SLEEP, EPILEPSIES, AND COGNITIVE IMPAIRMENT

SLEEP, EPILEPSIES, AND COGNITIVE IMPAIRMENT

PÉTER HALÁSZ

ANNA SZŰCS

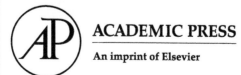

ACADEMIC PRESS

An imprint of Elsevier

Academic Press is an imprint of Elsevier
125 London Wall, London EC2Y 5AS, United Kingdom
525 B Street, Suite 1800, San Diego, CA 92101-4495, United States
50 Hampshire Street, 5th Floor, Cambridge, MA 02139, United States
The Boulevard, Langford Lane, Kidlington, Oxford OX5 1GB, United Kingdom

Library of Congress Cataloging-in-Publication Data
A catalog record for this book is available from the Library of Congress

British Library Cataloguing-in-Publication Data
A catalogue record for this book is available from the British Library

ISBN: 978-0-12-812579-3

For information on all Academic press publications visit our website at
https://www.elsevier.com/books-and-journals

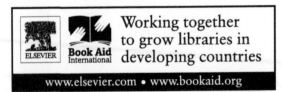

Working together
to grow libraries in
developing countries

www.elsevier.com • www.bookaid.org

Publisher: Nikki Levy
Acquisition Editor: Melanie Tucker
Editorial Project Manager: Kathy Padilla
Production Project Manager: Anusha Sambamoorthy
Designer: Mark Rogers

Typeset by TNQ Books and Journals

Contents

3. Autosomal Dominant Nocturnal Frontal Lobe and Nocturnal Frontal Lobe Epilepsy as System Epilepsies of the Ascending Cholinergic Arousal System

4. Juvenile Idiopathic Myoclonic Epilepsy (Janz Syndrome) as a System Epilepsy Affecting the Corticothalamic System and the Frontal Motor and Cognitive Frontal Subsystems

5. Medial Temporal Lobe Epilepsy (MTLE): The Epilepsy of the Hippocampal Declarative Memory System

6. Idiopathic Polyfocal Hyperexcitability Conditions (HIEC) of Childhood and Their Transition to Electrical Status Epilepticus in Sleep

7. Epileptic Encephalopathies

8. Summary

Index

Acknowledgments

We would like to express our warm thanks to our colleagues for shaping our approach and learning from one another during the years we spent together as a team, first in the National Institute of Psychiatry and Neurology and then in the National Institute of Clinical Neurosciences and in other collaborations, which, it is hoped, we have all enjoyed:

Acsádi László, Balogh Attila, Barcs Gábor, Barsi Péter, Bódizs Róbert, Borbély Csaba, Clemens Béla, Clemens Zsófia, Fabó Dániel, Fehér Ottó, Fogarasi András, György Ilona, Hegyi Márta, Holló András, Janszky József, Juhos Vera, Jerney Judit, Kelemen Anna, Köves Péter, Maglóczky Zsófia, Rajna Péter, Rásonyi György, Siegler Zsuzsa, Szente Magdolna, Szűcs Anna, Újma Péter, Ujszászi János, and Ulbert István.

Péter Halász is grateful to those researchers with high international reputations, from whom he could learn a great deal and whose thoughts have inspired him:

Alexander Borbély, Jan Colrain, Guis Declerck, Allan Hobson, Georg Kostopoulos, Michel Koutroumanidis, Lino Nobili, Liborio Parrino, Piere Passouant, Lopez da Silva, Carlo Alberto Tassinari, Mario Terzano, and Peter Wolf.

We received much help in the editing, and language and spelling correction, of this book from several young colleagues, especially Ákos Újvári, Márta Virág, and Zsófia Jordán, for which we are also deeply grateful. We are grateful for the work of Dr. Julia Gádoros (wife of Péter Halász): she has given continuous help during the preparation of this book concerning both theoretical and technical issues.

Owing to the nature of our work, the diagnostic and treatment activity is strongly interwoven with scientific research for better understanding of the disease; so our patients had an important part in this work. We are thankful to them for the opportunity to work with them.

We are grateful for the support of the National Brain Research Program (KTIA_NAP_13-1-2013-0001).

Author Profiles

DR. PÉTER HALÁSZ

Péter Halász is an Emeritus Professor of Neurology, PhD, DSCi, working in epileptology and sleep research.

He has published several books and book chapters and more than 200 peer-reviewed papers about various epilepsy and sleep-related topics. He was the first president of the Hungarian Sleep Society and the founder of the Hungarian Epilepsy League and of the Hungarian Epilepsy Surgery Program and was the head for several years of the Hungarian Comprehensive Epilepsy Center. He was honored for his international activity by the International League Against Epilepsy with the title "Ambassador of Epilepsy."

He has extensive experience in postgraduate education and worldwide teaching in issues of epilepsy and sleep and works regularly as a reviewer for several international journals.

DR. ANNA SZŰCS

Anna Szűcs is a clinical neurologist and psychiatrist with several fields of interest. She started work as a psychiatrist, and then, for a long time, worked as a neurologist, while also specializing in sleep medicine and epileptology. She has experience in the presurgical electrophysiological evaluation of epileptic patients and in the chronic care of patients living with epilepsy, having done numerous epilepsy and sleep clinic studies. She has worked as a consultant neurologist in the Neurology Department of the National Institute of Clinical Neurosciences, Budapest.

In addition to her practice in Hungary she has worked from time to time in the United Kingdom as a consultant in neurology since 2009 and has traveled to many areas, studying in several European departments and laboratories.

She has several international publications with an impact factor of 120 and a citation index of about 600. She has written books and book chapters on narcolepsy, sleep disorders, and selected fields of epileptology. She has a PhD, habilitated in neurology in 2010.

She has been working with Professor Halász since 1994.

Glossary

ACh Acetylcholine
ADNFLE Autosomal dominant nocturnal frontal lobe epilepsy
Atypical rolandic epilepsy Rolandic epilepsy transforming toward ESES/Landau–Kleffner syndrome
APs Arousal parasomnias
BCTE spikes Benign centrotemporal epilepsy spikes
BOLD Blood oxygen level–dependent MRI response
CAE Childhood absence epilepsy
CAP Cyclic alternating pattern in sleep EEG
CAP A phase A (phasic activation)-type cyclic alternating pattern
CAP A1-A2-A3 CAP A phase subtypes
CAP B phase B (background)-type cyclic alternating pattern
DC Direct current
DMN Default mode network
DTI Diffusion tensor imaging (imaging brain pathways with magnetic resonance)
EEG Electroencephalography
EEG–fMRI EEG-based functional magnetic resonance imaging
EEs Epileptic encephalopathies
ESES Electrical status epilepticus in sleep
FCD Focal cortical dysplasia
FDG–PET Fluorodeoxyglucose PET
FO electrode Foramen ovale electrode
GABA Gamma-butyric acid (inhibitory neurotransmitter of gap junction)
GOE Late-onset childhood benign occipital epilepsy
GPFA Generalized paroxysmal fast activity
GTCS Generalized tonic–clonic seizure
HFO High-frequency oscillation
HIEC Hyperexcitability condition
HS Hippocampal sclerosis
Hypsarrhythmia Chaotic mixture of spikes and slow waves in West syndrome
IEDs Interictal epileptiform discharges
IGE Idiopathic generalized epilepsy
IPN Interpeduncular nucleus
JAE Juvenile absence epilepsy
JME Juvenile myoclonic epilepsy (Janz syndrome)
LDT Laterodorsal tegmental nucleus
LGS Lennox–Gastaut syndrome
LTP Long-term potentiation
MRI Magnetic resonance imaging
MTLE Medial temporal lobe epilepsy
mTOR Mechanistic target of rapamycin
nAChR Nicotinic acetylcholine receptor
NFLE Nocturnal frontal lobe epilepsy
NMDA *N*-methyl-D-aspartate

NREM Non-REM sleep
Ohtahara syndrome Early infantile epileptic encephalopathy
PET Positron emission tomography
PS Panayiotopoulos syndrome (early-onset benign occipital seizure susceptibility)
RE Thalamic reticular nucleus
REM Rapid eye movement (sleep)
Rolandic epilepsy Childhood benign focal epilepsy with centrotemporal spikes
SHE Sleep-related hypermotor epilepsy
SMA Supplementary motor area
SPECT Single photon emission tomography
SPW-r Sharp wave–ripple
SWD Bilateral synchronous spike–wave discharge
SWS Slow-wave sleep
TC Thalamocortical neuron
TCI Transient cognitive impairment
TLE Temporal lobe epilepsy
West syndrome Epileptic encephalopathy with hypsarrhythmia and infantile spasms

Preface

This book brings a fresh outlook on epilepsy syndromes. Péter Halász and Anna Szűcs call this an unorthodox approach. Rightly so! It is refreshing to read a book in which the basic concepts of epilepsies are presented in an unconventional way, beyond the classic dichotomy—"focal versus generalized"—highlighting the importance of considering the links between the noticeable vulnerability of some networks of the brain to epileptic manifestations, on the one hand, and their capacity to exhibit conspicuous dynamic features of neural plasticity, on the other.

Two systems stand out in this context: one consists of the corticothalamic networks that exert control over sleep and wakefulness and regulate the homeostatic balance of synaptic loads and the formation of memory traces; the other is the system formed by the hippocampal and associated cortical networks that play a predominant role in plastic changes at the network, cellular, and molecular levels necessary for memory formation and consolidation.

Plastic systems are inherently dynamic. It is a general characteristic of complex dynamic systems that changes in parameters, whether intrinsic or associated with extrinsic stimuli, can lead to the occurrence of unstable behavior, which ultimately can cause sudden transitions between dynamic states; in the case of brain systems this implies the transition between a normal state and an epileptic state. The latter is characterized by abnormal oscillations and typical behavioral manifestations. This is essentially what happens, in general, when epileptic seizures occur.

The authors point out in a convincing way that epilepsy should be considered a *derailment of brain plastic functions*. In other words it may be considered a consequence of changes in some parameters of neuronal networks that under normal limits display strong plastic properties, but if those limits are exceeded a vulnerable network emerges, which, now and then, can display epileptic seizures. Along this basic line of thought the authors provide useful insights into a number of epileptic syndromes.

The derailment of brain plastic processes comes to the fore in a most dramatic form in the case of epilepsies of early onset related to epileptic encephalopathies. These disturb the development of neuronal networks not only at the cortical level but also at the level of cortico–subcortical association systems, where abnormal epileptic activity may affect synaptic formation and pruning, leading to the development of abnormal patterns of connectivity in the brain. This is, of course, of paramount relevance to understanding how cognitive impairments are associated with these forms of epilepsy syndromes.

The emphasis on dynamic aspects of epilepsy spreads throughout the whole book, and replaces the classic rigid dichotomy of "generalized" versus "focal" epilepsies. In absence epilepsy the classic "generalized" connotation can now be accounted for by the finding that specific cortical networks act as drivers of spike-and-wave discharges, which propagate very quickly bilaterally through the corticothalamic system; the classic "focal" epilepsies are not strictly bound to a circumscribed region either, rather the epileptic activity can involve more or less widespread networks, sometimes bilateral homologous regions (as in occipital and temporal lobe epilepsies).

Particularly original is the authors' approach regarding *sleep-related epilepsies*, namely absence epilepsy, as a form of systems epilepsy of the non–rapid eye movement (NREM) sleep-promoting functions, and frontal lobe epilepsies, resulting from abnormal dynamics of the arousal system arising from sleep. This is especially relevant taking into consideration the long-standing contributions of the authors to the field of sleep research, especially with respect to their approach to studying the dynamics of sleep oscillations in the framework of microstructural analysis of sleep. An interesting illustration of this approach is the way the authors relate the sleep-regulating role of arousals in the framework of the microcyclicity of sleep, i.e., the phases of the cyclic alternating pattern (CAP), with respect to epileptic events in absence epilepsies and in nocturnal frontal lobe epilepsy (NFLE), including the autosomal dominant type (ADNFLE). Patients with this syndrome carry gain-of-function mutations of the cholinergic nicotinic receptor subunits expressed mainly in the thalamus and other networks of the ascending arousal cholinergic system, which projects to the prefrontal cortex. In the CAP the activation of microshifts toward arousal or REM sleep (called A3 phase) alternates with microshifts in the opposite direction toward NREM sleep or antiarousal (A1 phase), depending on the level of homeostatic pressure. The authors showed that in ADNFLE patients, who have an activated cholinergic arousal system owing to the aforementioned mutation, epileptic events occur that are particularly associated with the arousal CAP A3 phase, whereas in absences such events occur preferentially associated with the NREM sleep CAP A1 phase. In this way it can be shown that ADNFLE (and also NFLE) and absences are two disorders of two antagonistic thalamocortical systems that control sleep and wakefulness. These findings highlight the train of thought that percolates through the whole book, namely the importance of understanding the tight relationship between the functional state of networks controlling vigilance/sleep and the likelihood of the occurrence of epileptic events. This line of reasoning extends further to the realm of the pathophysiology of arousal parasomnias (APs), putting into evidence the parallelism between APs and NFLE. The typical NFLE seizures are sometimes described as "movement storms" or "hypermotor seizures" but may present a variety of behavioral manifestations. The symptoms of APs are similar but, in general, more severe, and may take, for example, the form of "night terrors." Both conditions, NFLE and APs, share a common relation with sleep dynamics. To understand the underlying pathophysiology, with its similarities between NFLE and APs, it is important to realize that sleep is not a unitary phenomenon, as it was considered previously. Indeed regional sleep may coexist along awake states: this can account for the existence of dissociated states, what may explain automatic responses to environmental events, such as APs. The authors suggest that the common pathophysiological feature of NFLE and APs may be a dissociation of the prefrontal cortex from the rest of the cortex, underlying the loss of conscious control over the autonomic symptoms characteristic of both awakening related conditions. As the authors insightfully point out, the "epileptic automatisms and the supposed underlying dissociative mechanisms should move from the group of curiosities to be considered important factors of epileptic seizure semiology."

The book also gives a comprehensive analysis of medial temporal lobe epilepsy (MTLE), envisaged as an epilepsy of the hippocampal declarative memory system. In this connection special attention is given to the causal role of sharp waves (SPWs)–ripples in assisting learning and memory consolidation, particularly during NREM sleep; SPWs are phase modulated by sleep spindles and by the slow oscillation (<1 Hz). These hippocampal EEG phenomena play a role in the protection of memory engrams during the consolidation process. The authors point out that the SPW–ripple complex is at the "edge of the shift toward epileptic excitation," which would account for the vulnerability of the hippocampal system to the occurrence of epileptic activity. In this way the authors extend their argument that "epilepsy is a derailment of physiological functioning" also to MTLEs. Furthermore, on the basis of a short review of relevant literature, they refer to experimental evidence that the rate of SPW–ripples in epileptic patients during sleep decreases as the rate of epileptiform spikes increases, and draw the conclusion that "epileptic spiking contributes more to the memory disturbances in MTLE than we had expected."

In addition the authors dedicate the last chapters to an overview of the most common genetically determined nonlesional age-dependent childhood epilepsies, stressing the polyfocal hyperexcitability (HIEC) character of these conditions to indicate the occurrence of polyregional interictal epileptiform activities. Further, they review the conditions of the transformation of HIEC to electrical status epilepticus in sleep (ESES) and pay special attention to epileptic encephalopathies, such as the Landau–Kleffner syndrome (LKS) and West syndrome, also characterized by the involvement of sleep activation processes. With respect to these conditions, the authors propose the concept of the "perisylvian epileptic network" to account for benign focal childhood epilepsies that can transform into malignant encephalopathies, such as LKS or ESES. They stress the likelihood that these conditions may be related genetic variants displaying different phenotypes, with the common feature of the propensity for interictal epileptiform activity to occur during sleep. This feature may account for the cognitive impairments that often affect these children. Interestingly, the presence of high-frequency oscillations appears to correlate with the severity of epileptic encephalopathies, which would also contribute to the cognitive impairment in these conditions. In general, EEG suppression–burst activity during the whole sleep time seen in neonatal encephalopathies, as well as the hypsarrhythmia typical of West syndrome, probably interferes with normal brain development.

In short, this book represents the culmination of decades of insightful clinical research by two authors, both having outstanding track records in the analysis of epileptic phenomena, particularly in relation to sleep–wakefulness cycles.

This a scholarly book that presents a collection of innovative views and provocative ideas, anchored in a combination of extensive experience and deep scientific scrutiny.

Fernando H. Lopes da Silva, MD, PhD
Emeritus Professor
Center for Neuroscience, Swammerdam Institute for Life Sciences
Science Park 904, 1098XH Amsterdam, The Netherlands

Introductory Considerations

Owing to important progress in epilepsy and sleep research during the past decades, converging evidence has accumulated on new aspects of the interrelationship between sleep and epilepsy. Both fields have been enriched by the observations of intracranial recordings performed on epileptic patients under presurgical evaluation.

Sleep research has realized that the amount of sleep spindles and slow waves during non–rapid eye movement (NREM) sleep is associated with cognitive functions. It has become clear that slow-wave homeostatic regulation connects with synaptic homeostasis, determining the synaptic capacity of the brain for learning and memory (Tononi and Cirelli, 2003). Therefore, the link between sleep and epilepsy has been recognized as a key factor in the mechanism of cognitive impairment in epilepsy.

Epilepsy has an unknown face hidden in sleep. It is impossible to conceive the pathophysiology of several epilepsies without incorporating up-to-date knowledge about slow-wave sleep (SWS). Our book is devoted to this aim: exploring and reinterpreting the role of sleep in epilepsy.

For introduction, we briefly summarize the changes in and new aspects of both sleep and epilepsy and their relationship.

THE GROWING KNOWLEDGE ABOUT THE LINK BETWEEN NON–RAPID EYE MOVEMENT SLEEP AND PLASTIC FUNCTIONS OF THE BRAIN

There are convincing data supporting that one of the main biological functions of SWS is fueling plasticity, of which epilepsy may be considered a severe derailment (exaggeration) (Vyazovskiy et al., 2000; Huber et al., 2006; Buzsáki, 2015).

From the sleep side, our view of SWS has importantly changed. We consider sleep as a self-regulating open system in an organic interrelationship with both environmental stimuli and epileptic events, gating them by the elements of sleep microstructure. Understanding how different sleep constituents participate in cognitive functioning may shed light on the interference caused by epileptic events.

Since the 1970s a new, finer-graded sleep EEG analysis has developed beyond the broader frame of sleep states, established by Dement and Kleitman and elaborated in the form of a standardized scoring system by Rechtschaffen and Kales (1968).

The recognition of the finer-grade sleep structure and its dynamic nature started with the identification of recurring transient (phasic) events within the sleep EEG. The universal recurrence of phasic events in NREM sleep and the fact that they could be elicited by different stimuli highlighted that even seemingly spontaneous episodes might be evoked by unnoticed internal (within the body or brain) or environmental stimuli (Halász et al., 1979) not awakening the sleeper. Although the potential to elicit a phasic event proved to be variable by different stimulus modalities (acoustic stimuli prevail), the essential observation was the modality independence of these events. Another basic feature is the association with a variable degree of autonomic activation as heart rate and motor augmentation evidenced by EMG.

Whatever the input is, the reactive events belong to two types (Fig. 1.1). The first type behaves as a classical arousal response: an increase in the EEG frequency and a decrease in the amplitude. It is the "phases d'activation transitoire" (PAT) (Schieber et al., 1971) prototype. The second type is more sleep- than arousal-like, associated with no or lower intensity autonomic and motor changes. The EEG morphology is consistent with this sleep-like character: K complexes and slow-wave groups. During the 1970s and 1980s,

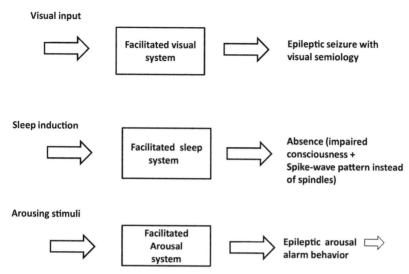

FIGURE 1.1 Working mode schemes of reflex epilepsies (top), system epilepsies of arousal (nocturnal frontal lobe epilepsy; bottom), and sleep induction (absence epilepsy; middle). System epilepsies are triggered by the operation of a system ignited by the specific sensory input. The intrinsic activation of the network of a physiologic system (such as the sleep or arousal system) also may result in system-specific epileptic manifestations if the given system has an increased susceptibility to epilepsy (see more details in Chapters 2 and 3).

it became clear that there is a continuous sleep level oscillation in each stage of NREM sleep, related to phasic events. We started to call them micro-arousals (Halász et al., 1979).

After the recognition of the "cyclic alternating pattern" (CAP) by the Parma Sleep Research Group (Terzano et al., 1985) a new microstructure broadened our dynamic view of NREM sleep (Fig. 1.2). The CAP is a microcyclicity: present during all NREM sleep stages and constituted by alternations of activated (A phase) and background (B phase) periods. According to the type of activation in phase A, three categories (Fig. 1.3) have been differentiated (Terzano et al., 2000): (1) Phase A1 exclusively comprises K complexes and slow waves, functionally representing an "antiarousal," i.e., a shift toward sleep. (2) Phase A3 is an arousal pattern with attenuated fast activity and muscle and autonomic arousal signs. It is identical with the PAT pattern, and the arousals are recognized by the ASDA (1990). (3) Phase 2 is an intermediate, mixed pattern, usually starting with slow waves and turning to a faster desynchronized activity.

The descending (D) and ascending (A) slopes of the sleep cycles show opposite trends (Fig. 1.3). Slope D carries sleep-promoting, whereas slope A presents wake/rapid eye movement (REM)-promoting tendencies. The arousal-like phasic changes (CAP A 2–3 phases) turned out to dominate

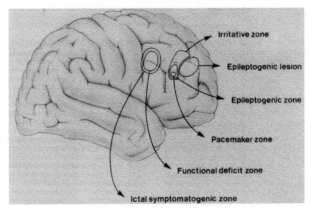

- Epileptogenic lesion   Neuroimaging, neuropathology
- Irritative zone   Interictal EEG (IEDs and HFO)
- Pacemaker zone   Ictal invasive EEG (ictal EEG and HFO)
- Symptomatogenic zone   Video-EEG with testing
- Functional deficit zone   EEG, interictal SPECT, PET, MRspectroscopy

FIGURE 1.2 Top: The Lüders–Awad epileptic zones [*epileptic lesion*, the epileptogenic structural lesion; *irritative zone*, the interictal spiking area; *pacemaker zone*, seizure onset zone; *symptomatogenic zone*, the region producing the first detected seizure symptom; *functional deficit zone*, the region of the interictal (or postparoxysmal) deficit symptoms]. Bottom: Diagnostic methods for detecting the epileptic zones. *HFO*, high-frequency oscillation; *IEDs*, interictal epileptic discharges; *PET*, positron emission tomography; *SPECT*, single photon emission computed tomography.

the A slopes of the sleep cycles, and their occurrence increases from evening to morning. Within the A slopes, their prevalence is higher before the REM sleep periods. The sleep-like phasic changes (the slow waves of CAP A1) have a reverse course. They are prevalent during the D slopes of the night's first sleep cycles and follow the homeostatic decay of slow-wave oscillation both within one cycle and from cycle to cycle. The two types of phasic events have opposite tendencies during the night sleep from evening to morning: whereas the arousal-like responses tend to increase, the sleep-like responses tend to decrease (Halász and Bódizs, 2013).

This distribution seems to clearly follow the interplay of sleep- and wake/REM-promoting forces both within the individual cycles and through the whole night course, probably in association with the interactions of reciprocal antagonistic brain stem networks determining cortical responsiveness (Takahashi et al., 2010) (Fig. 1.4). Therefore, CAP episodes are microstructural elements of sleep, exemplifying that microstates build up macrostates.

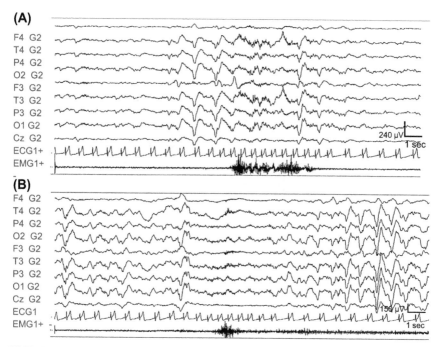

FIGURE 1.3   Two types of non–rapid eye movement sleep responses to sensory stimulation: type *A*, sleep-like (antiarousal) response with K complexes and slow waves with autonomic—heart rate and muscle—activation [identical with cyclic alternating pattern (CAP) A1 phase], and type *B*, amplitude attenuation with fast waves, autonomic and muscle activation consistent with the classical arousal response (identical with CAP A3 and with "microarousals from sleep") of the American Sleep Disorders Association.

To summarize the significance of the CAP:

The CAP subtypes as responses to external or internal stimuli indicate the level of the actual sleep propensity across the night sleep.

NREM sleep is an open system reacting to changes in the environment. The CAP is an indicator of physiological and pathological sleep instability and it has a role in marking out (gating) pathological sleep events (Parrino et al., 2000).

The homeostatic aspects of the CAP show how external influences fuel reactive slow-wave activity necessary for sleep plastic functioning (Halász et al., 2014).

External influences participate in sleep regulation (Halász, Bódizs, 2013).

The knowledge about homeostatic regulation has gained important new connotations. Homeostatic regulation in general is the control and maintenance of a stable and constant condition, achieved usually by a negative feedback mechanism. NREM sleep is controlled by the homeostatic process; this is measurably expressed by slow-wave activity (SWA). Sleep loss leads to a proportional increase in SWA (0.75–4.5 Hz) during the

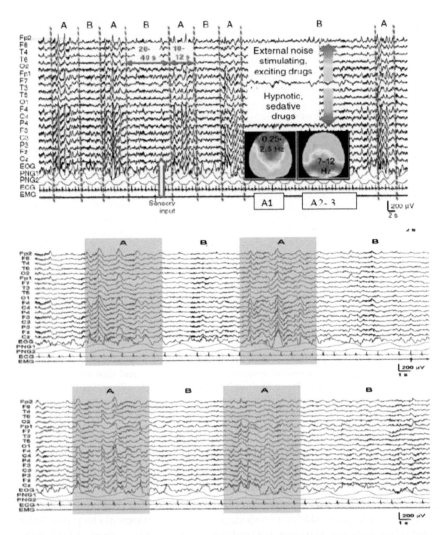

FIGURE 1.4 Electromorphological elements of cyclic alternating pattern (CAP) A and B phases, their time relations, and their reactability. The inset diagrams show the CAP subtypes power spectrum distribution over the scalp (see more detail in the text). The CAP rate increases in reaction to sleep-disturbing sensory inputs, to stimulatory drugs; it decreases under hypnotic drugs. *Empty arrow*, acoustic stimuli applied during phase B, eliciting phase A.

next sleep. Sleep propensity exponentially increases during the waking state from morning to evening, whereas the power of SWA exponentially decreases from evening to morning. In line with this slow-wave decline, the capacity for learning and memory increases. Sleep loss is associated with cognitive impairment and the feeling of "sleepiness" (Horne and Wilkinson, 1985; Borbély, 1982; Dijk et al., 1987; Achermann et al., 1995).

Since the beginning of the 21st century, the local aspects of homeo-static regulation have received increasing attention. The frontal prepon-derance of sleep SWA as well as the frontal and dominant hemisphere excess of the recovery increase in slow waves after sleep deprivation has been demonstrated (Cajochen et al., 1999; Marzano et al., 2010, Achermann et al., 2001; Finelli et al., 2001). Extensive sensory stimula-tion of one hand prior to sleep led to an increase in sleep delta power in the opposite hemisphere over the somatosensory arm area (Kattler et al., 1994) and the inverse: the immobilization of the arm caused a local reduction in delta power in the same area (Huber et al., 2006). The effect of cutting the whiskers of rats on one side was similar, regard-ing changes in hemispheric asymmetry in their sleep SWA (Vyazovskiy et al., 2000).

When learning and synaptic plasticity were related to sleep SWA, the notion of experience dependency emerged, suggesting that it is the net change in synaptic strength that is important for sleep homeostasis (Tononi and Cirelli, 2003).

Therefore, there is convincing evidence supporting that use-dependent plasticity processes (Kattler et al., 1994; Huber et al., 2006; Vyazovskiy et al., 2000) govern NREM sleep, especially SWS homeostatic regulation. In other words, slow-wave homeostasis and use-dependent plasticity are two sides of the same coin representing the biological function of SWS. The full-blown evolution of this complex regulation is probably a human neoformation related to high cognitive functions and the consequent vul-nerability of the frontal neocortex.

Thus, the concept of sleep homeostatic regulation has importantly changed. The empty envelope of the interrelationship between the dura-tion of wakefulness and the slow-wave content of the consecutive sleep period has been filled up with a neurophysiological content. SWS has been endowed with a new role: refreshing the synaptic connections oversatu-rated during the daytime, allowing them to regain their learning capacity for the next day.

The conceptual changes of sleep homeostatic regulation are summa-rized in Table 1.1.

The first recognized example of reactive slow waves was the K com-plex (KC), a characteristic spontaneous constituent of stage 2 NREM sleep (Halász, 2005). Its elicitation by acoustic stimuli (it can also be evoked by other sensory stimuli) was described at the beginning of the sleep EEG era. Loomis (Loomis et al., 1937), probably the first systematic sleep elec-troencephalographer, recognized that knocking on the sleeper's room door elicits a huge biphasic bilateral frontal slow wave, hence the name "K complex."

Three reviews provide a broad overview of 70 years of history and inter-pretations of this sleep graphoelement (Colrain, 2005; Halász, 2005, 2015).

TABLE 1.1   Changing Views About Sleep Homeostasis

Theoretical Framework	Nature of Sleep Homeostasis	Key Factor in Sleep Homeostasis	Experimental Protocol	Neurochemical Background (Antecedents)	Key References
Two-process model	Sleep–wake dependent	Presleep wakefulness	Constant routine	Hypnotoxin theory	Borbély et al. (1981); Borbély (1982)
Neuronal group theory	Use dependent	Afferent stimulation	Presleep stimulation	Somnogenic cytokines	Krueger and Obál (1993); Kattler et al. (1994)
Synaptic homeostasis	Experience dependent	Learning	Presleep learning	Long-term potentiation-related neurochemical factors	Tononi and Cirelli (2003); Huber et al. (2006)

The components of the KC, an evoked response during NREM sleep, and its topographical features have been scrutinized as well (Ujszászi and Halász, 1988; Bastien et al., 2002). The pattern could also be detected by averaging techniques in deep sleep, where its spontaneous appearance is not easily captured.

The relationship of the KC with the slow-wave oscillation (<1 Hz) was clarified by Amzica and Steriade in the 1990s and later by Cash et al. (2009). The similarity of the large negative main component of the KC with the down state of slow oscillation is the most important argument supporting their fundamental identity (Fig. 1.5).

The elicitation of the CAP A1 (antiarousal) pattern by acoustic stimuli during CAP B phases has proven that a certain amount of (reactive) sleep slow waves (probably those with the highest amplitudes and the strongest synchrony) are evoked by sensory stimulation, as also confirmed by elegant experiments (Riedner et al., 2011; Laurino et al., 2014).

Further proofs for the reactive slow-wave phenomenon were provided by the artificial boosting of slow waves by transcranial magnetic stimulation (Massimini et al., 2007), transcranial electrical stimulation

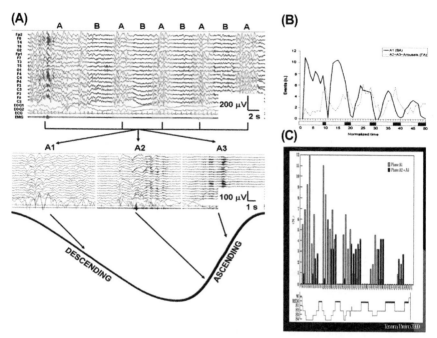

FIGURE 1.5 (A) The distribution of the three subtypes of cyclic alternating pattern (CAP) A phase—A1, A2, A3—across the sleep cycle. Increased homeostatic pressure promotes CAP A1; decreasing homeostatic pressure is associated with A2 and low homeostatic pressure with A3. (B) The distribution of CAP A subtypes across the night sleep: A1 follows the dampening course of homeostatic pressure from evening to morning; A2 and A3 increase and peak before rapid eye movement (*REM*) sleep in each cycle. (C) Detailed distributions of CAP A1, A2, and A3 phases on the descending and ascending slopes of sleep cycles: A1 dominates the first two cycles and the descending slopes of the cycles, whereas A2 and A3 prevail during the last third of the night and the ascending slopes of the cycles.

(Vyazovskiy et al., 2009), and acoustic stimulation (Ngo et al., 2013; Bellesi et al., 2014). Besides single reactive slow waves, a stepwise deepening of sleep has developed in reaction to the stimulation; suggesting that NREM sleep can be entrained by external stimuli.

We proposed that CAP phase A1 represents a slow-wave "injection," supplementing the necessary amount of slow waves during sleep. Thus, when any sleep-disturbing external influences threaten with a drop of slow waves below a critical level, an extra production of slow waves ensures protection for the vulnerable human frontal lobe. This would be an "instant homeostatic regulation" on top of the traditional one with a longer time constant, working in the next sleep period. This instant regulation works during the very night in which the interfering

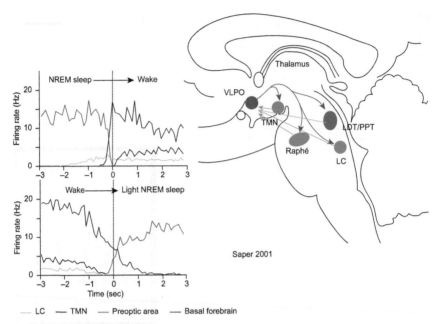

FIGURE 1.6   Right: The reciprocal inhibitory relationship of the hypothalamic ventro-lateral preoptic nucleus (*VLPO*) sleep system (red arrows) and the brain stem ascending reticular arousal system (green arrow) with subsystems using different transmitters (based on Saper's work 2001; modified). Left: The unit discharge frequency in different wake-promoting and basal forebrain (*preoptic area* and *basal forebrain* nuclei) sleep-promoting areas in non–rapid eye movement (*NREM*)–wakefulness (top) and wakefulness–NREM (bottom) transition periods (based on Takahashi's work). *LC*, locus coeruleus (adrenergic); *LDT/PPT*, laterodorsal tegmental/pedunculopontine nuclei (cholinergic); *Raphé*, Raphe nucleus (serotoninergic); *TMN*, tuberomammillary nucleus (histaminergic).

disturbance occurs. Thus, the human frontal lobe is under a "double helmet" protecting the newly developed human frontal lobe functions (Fig. 1.6).

CHANGING CONCEPTUAL FRAMEWORKS IN EPILEPSY

Epilepsies as Disorders of Neural Plasticity

From the epilepsy side, there is growing evidence that the common feature underlying epileptic mechanisms, in general, is a derailment of dynamic plastic changes. This concept explains the ubiquity of epilepsy in the animal world and its high prevalence among brain disorders, anchoring in cortical, corticothalamic, and archicortical (hippocampal) brain structures, the substrates of plastic changes. The consistently accepted idea is that epilepsy is a chronically raised state of excitability affecting certain cortical structures, enabling them to generate interictal epileptiform discharges (IEDs) and seizures. Buzsáki (1986) remembered the work of Goddard and Douglas (1975). He was the first to propose that the plastic changes of long-term potentiation and kindling epileptogenesis may involve similar processes (Goddard 1983) Repetitive stimuli may generate physiological long-term potentiation (LTP) resulting in learning, whereas during epileptic kindling, repetitive stimulation leads to afterdischarges and seizures. In rats hippocampal kindling impairs working and long-term memory (reviewed in Gorter et al., (2016).

Terje Lomo and Timothy Bliss discovered LTP in 1966 in the rabbit hippocampus (Bliss and Lomo, 1973). They stimulated the perforant path of the hippocampus—proceeding to the dentate gyrus—and registered the response (excitatory postsynaptic potential; EPSP). If they applied a serial stimulation, the subsequent stimulus evoked a longer lasting and larger amplitude EPSP and the elevated responsivity was permanent (lasted longer). A forerunner of LTP was elaborated by Donald Hebb, inspired by the fundamental studies of Ramon y Cajal published as early as in 1894, who used the term "plasticity" to describe his findings regarding degeneration and regeneration phenomena in the nervous system (Stahnisch and Nitsch 2002).

Hebb supposed that, in the course of repeated stimulation, the presynaptic neuron induces some kinds of growth and metabolic changes in the postsynaptic neuron. The physical and biological bases of this phenomenon are still the object of intense scrutiny. We know that LTP is associated with the increase in the number of postsynaptic receptors and synaptic transmitters resulting in the strengthening of some intercellular connections.

The contradictions around the dichotomic views of focal/regional and generalized epilepsies have necessitated finding new conceptual frameworks for epilepsy classification. This has required the practical use of the brain network concept to epilepsy (Avanzini et al., 2012), using up-to-date functional and imaging methods for investigating brain connectivity.

Epilepsies as Network Disorders

The concept of epileptic networks provides a new framework for the understanding of nonlesional "idiopathic" and lesional epilepsies involving widespread brain systems. The network concept and the term "system epilepsy" are more or less overlapping ideas. The essential feature of the latter is the endeavor linking epilepsy to existing brain networks/systems (Avanzini et al., 2012; Capovilla et al., 2013; Wolf et al., 2015). According to this concept, epilepsy, especially if it starts

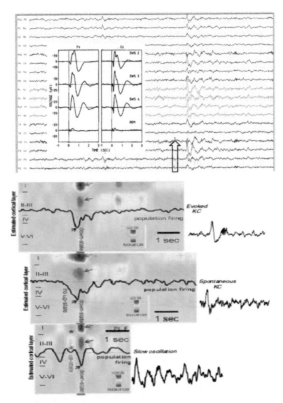

FIGURE 1.7 Spontaneous and evoked K complexes (*KC*) in stage 2 non–rapid eye movement (NREM) sleep and comparison with spontaneous slow activity, both detected by multilayer laminar microwire electrodes (cortical layers are indicated on the left side). The down states of spontaneous and evoked K complexes seem to be identical with slow-wave down states based on the situation of sinks and sources by the current source density method (modified from Cash et al., 2009, with permission). Left: Averaged K complexes of 10 healthy young persons over the Fz and Cz electrodes during NREM sleep (*SWS*) stages 2–4 and rapid eye movement (*REM*) sleep.

early, would use or "hijack" the "templates" of big physiologic systems (Beenhakker and Huguenard, 2009).

In between the static geometrical concept of the site of epileptic dysfunction linked to a "focus" and the idea of an epilepsy network, the epileptic zones model of Lüders and Awad (Lüders and Awad, 1992;Rosenow and Lüders, 2001) has represented an advancement (Fig. 1.7) providing a more differentiated spatial distribution of epilepsy-related regions. This model identifies the "epileptogenic lesion" underlying the epilepsy, the interictal spiking zone referred to as "irritative," and the seizure-initiating or pacemaker zone, while the region responsible for the clinical symptoms is the "symptomatogenic" or "executive" zone. The hypothetical zone called

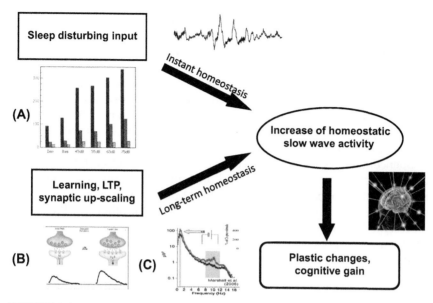

FIGURE 1.8   Schematic composition showing the increasing effect on homeostatic slow-wave activity by both traditional long-term and (newly described) instant homeostatic regulation. (A) Selective increase in cyclic alternating pattern (*CAP*) A1 rate following the loudness of the acoustic stimulation during stage 2 non–rapid eye movement sleep compared to other CAP subtypes (columns with decreasing intensity). (B) Long-term potentiation (*LTP*) increase by potentiation of the postsynaptic depolarization response to repetitive stimulation of the presynaptic nerve. This is a model of long-term homeostatic changes after boosting slow-wave activity by transcranial electrical simulation (C).

"epileptogenic" can be identified just a posteriori: only the outcome of the surgical intervention can show whether the size of the resected region was necessary and sufficient for seizure freedom. This model has provided standardized frameworks for the complex topographical and time relations of interictal and ictal events; however, it has not explicitly considered them. It has maintained the focal/generalized dichotomy focusing just on focal and surgically treatable epilepsies.

The understanding of the system idea may be helped by going back to "reflex epilepsies," considered unique, particular phenomena earlier (Fig. 1.8). The mechanism of reflex epilepsy involves the epileptic facilitation of a functional (typically sensory or sensorimotor) brain system. Stimulation of the peripheral afferents involving the system activates the epileptic manifestations. A good example is occipital visual system epilepsy, triggered by light stimuli across the activation of the epileptically facilitated occipital cortex. There are several papers on epilepsies evoked by additional stimuli, e.g., mental tasks, physical activities, cognitive or emotional triggers (Wolf, 2015), and also in cases underlain by brain lesions. Depending on the function of the facilitated structure, music, certain movements, reading, or playing chess or cards may become "epileptogenic"; any intervention specifically activating a brain region with epileptic susceptibility may evoke seizures. In the system epilepsy concept, we extend the mechanism of reflex epilepsies to any functional networks (brain systems): the activation of the network function may elicit the epileptic activity embedded in the given network. Finally, not an external stimulation itself, but network activation is the epileptogenic trigger, e.g., sleep-related epilepsies ignited by sleep induction or arousal (see Chapters 2 and 3).

Spencer (2002) was the first to define the epileptic network from a clinical perspective: "a functionally and anatomically connected, bilaterally represented set of cortical and subcortical brain structures and regions in which activity in any one part affects activity in all the others." ("Bilaterally represented" is now somewhat dubious.)

The most important argument supporting the network concept is the nature of epileptic dysfunction itself. Epilepsy "occupies" physiologically important structures of a sophisticated spatial network involving distant brain structures. The epileptic facilitation of the affected regions renders them sensitive (susceptible to seizing) in reaction to the incoming impulses. In other words, it is likely that a widespread network beyond the narrow seizure onset zone determines epilepsy; it is not restricted to circumscribed anatomical structures, but rather to functional brain systems.

During invasive presurgical investigations the involved structures outline a spatial network; in this respect it is relevant to note the relations between these structures and the occurrence of high-frequency oscillations (HFOs) as well (Jacobs et al., 2010, Jefferys et al., 2012, Haegelen et al., 2013, Höller et al., 2015, Jacobs et al., 2016).

EEG-based functional MRI (EEG–fMRI) is able to detect tissue oxygen consumption related to parallel registered EEG patterns. The fMRI with high resolution and spatial orientation can explore the link between brain structures, while the EEG detects functional features and measures their time relations. EEG–fMRI has been introduced into epilepsy research and has importantly contributed to the development of the epileptic network concept.

The results of spike-triggered EEG–fMRI studies support the network concept (Fahoum et al., 2012; Pittau et al., 2012). In the preictal/ictal period of temporal lobe seizures both positive and negative blood oxygen level–dependent (BOLD) responses appeared over the temporal lobes and in extratemporal structures as well, awaiting further clarification.

Gotman et al. (2005) from the Montreal Neurological Institute published a series of important results about BOLD changes during interictal and ictal epileptic EEG discharges. First, they revealed that the interictal spike discharges show several distant BOLD changes in addition to the local BOLD activation, and some of both the local and the distant changes are BOLD negative. Thus, BOLD activation seems to highlight a broader and more complex network of the spike discharges than we had expected.

Underlying the bilateral synchronous spike–wave discharges, a peculiar network has shown up. In accordance with the electrophysiological results of Steriade (2003) this network was found to be characterized by thalamic BOLD positive and a diffuse bilateral frontal dominant mosaic of mixed BOLD negative and positive spots with BOLD negative preponderance over the cortex (Fig. 2.6) (Aghakhani et al., 2004). The events identified as "secondary bilateral synchronization" have shown a similar diffuse bilateral BOLD negative-dominant mosaic cortical activation pattern (Aghakhani et al., 2006).

In certain seizures in which movement did not disturb the measurement an ictal BOLD activation could be detected, contributing to revealing the seizure onset and the propagation pattern as well.

With group analyses of the individual interictal BOLD changes in different types of epilepsies (temporal, frontal lobe, and posterior quadrant), Fahoum et al. (2012) from Gotman's group could demonstrate common metabolic changes shared by each type, which may remain undetected by imaging single patients during seizures.

Thus, the Gotman group has proposed that fMRI is a proper method for noninvasively mapping and three-dimensionally imaging both the interictal and (currently to a limited extent) the ictal network of epilepsy.

The reconsideration of reflex epilepsies also suggests the existence of widespread, interictal, and seizure-prone networks activated by specific stimuli (see for example the work of Meletti et al., 2016).

The development of pathologic networks in some forms of epilepsy should be considered in the general framework of the concepts of Hughlings Jackson, who conceived of the brain in a developmental hierarchy. Both the system and the spectrum aspects of epilepsy have strong implications fed by the developmental view.

Early-onset epilepsies related to epileptic encephalopathies distort the physiological functioning of corticocortical and cortico–subcortical association systems. Through deprogramming of the immature brain in epileptic encephalopathies, the epileptic variants of the physiological networks build up, as shown by contemporary imaging methods (EEG–fMRI, tensor imaging, receptor PET, etc.). This is well illustrated by the study of Chugani et al. (1992), who developed a network model to account for seizures and interictal phenomena in West syndrome using a special receptor PET investigation. They assumed that the epileptic discharges of a primary cortical epileptogenic lesion (e.g., a cortical dysplasia) would impinge on the serotonergic nuclei of the brain stem raphe, which in turn project pathological activity to the striatum and further on to the cortex; this would lead to the EEG hypsarrhythmia pattern. At the same time, descending impulses from the basal ganglia through the spinal tracts would cause bilateral spasms (Fig. 7.1).

Blume (2001) deduced the mechanism of Lennox–Gastaut syndrome from the excitability changes in cortical and thalamic structures resulting in pathologic activation patterns in the early phase of brain development, which is particularly vulnerable to this abnormal activity. Seizures may halt the remodeling of synaptic development, thus inhibiting pruning[1] and resulting in an overwired, "hyperconnective" brain, as is shown to occur in the somatosensory cortex of the rat (Navlakha et al., 2015). One of the mechanisms producing the pathological ties during early development is the elevation of neurotrophin levels by excitatory epileptic impulses that can lead to a pathologic increase in neuronal differentiation. The damage of some axons may influence the arborization of others, resulting in abnormal synaptic connections and adverse hyperconnectivity. Electric synapses (gap junctions[2]) may also contribute to pathological synchronization in early encephalopathies.

Of the two electroencephalographic aspects—ictal and interictal—of epilepsy, the ictal features usually attract more attention from clinicians, not only because a primary objective is that patients should be rid of seizures, but also because the emergence of surgical treatment led to a focus on defining the seizure onset zone, because the aim of surgery is to eliminate "seizures." Nowadays attention is given also to the interictal activity, in relation to both cognitive dysfunctions and sleep. In this book, we will pay special attention to the specific role of interictal spiking during SWS and its relation to cognitive dysfunction.

---

[1] The term "pruning" (cutting or section), originating from botany, describes the artificial shaping and cutting of plants. In cell biology, this term refers to a specific brain process, when nonfunctional, unused synapses and other neuronal elements waste away. In some forms of epilepsy, there is a failure of pruning as well as a failure of physiological differentiation. Epilepsy creates a hyperconnectivity of a given area, providing abundant epileptic discharges; it maintains a pathological functioning and inhibits pruning (as in hemimegalencephaly).

[2] Gap junction or "electric synapse" is a form of intercellular connection without chemical transmitters. The cytoplasms of two cells are directly linked, allowing the transfer of electrolytes, molecules, and electric impulses through a "gate" from one cell to the other. There are gap junctions in nearly every tissue. Gap junctions may have an important role in epileptic dysfunction and may contribute to the mechanism of HFOs, considered possible biomarkers of epilepsy (Tseng et al., 2008).

Epilepsies as Spectrum Disorders

The concept of system epilepsies and epileptic networks is quickly spreading in line with the notion of epilepsy being a "spectrum disorder," a term, first used in psychiatry, to indicate pathological conditions that do not constitute a unitary disorder, but rather a syndrome composed of diverse groups of symptoms (Jensen 2011). Spectrum diseases usually belong to a group of overlapping conditions (such as in cycloid personality traits, psychoses spectrum, obsessive–compulsive spectrum, and more recently "autism spectrum").

The developmental aspect is strong in the thinking about diseases of the nervous system since Hughlings Jackson, who conceived of the brain as a developmental hierarchy. Both the system and the spectrum aspects of epilepsy have strong implications fed by the developmental view. The essence of epileptic spectrum disorders, albeit named differently, was recognized in diverse types of genetic (idiopathic in the old terminology) generalized epilepsy. Indeed "endophenotypic" features are shared by different epileptic subtypes, such as the EEG patterns "bilateral synchronous spike–waves" and "centrotemporal spikes" (Fig. 6.5).

To understand the cognitive impairments associated with certain subtypes of the epilepsy spectrum of disorders it is important to realize that the brain executes hierarchically organized tasks during cognitive functioning. To understand this working mode, one needs to consider operational rules by which different brain areas cooperate. An important rule is that "parallel distributed processing" (see Mesulam, 1998) dominates the architecture of cognitive functions (as a counterpart of serial processing). The modules of the network contribute to the processing in flexible, changing combinations, without steady individual roles; rather the main thrust lies in the dynamics of variable coupling patterns of active networks. Another important principle is that functional binding of neuronal elements is realized by different oscillation frequencies that tend to synchronize in different combinations—these constitute the language of communication between networks of the functioning brain. Thus beyond spatial connectivity, time-related mechanisms called synchronization, coupling even distant brain regions, contribute importantly to cognitive brain functioning. In the presence of epileptic activities this functionally organized pattern of synchronized networks is disrupted, since epileptic excitation has a long-reaching impact on distant brain regions through the involved neuronal networks. These networks are characterized by the ability to convey epileptic abnormal activities and generate remote secondary epileptic conditions, while partially preserving their physiologic functional connections ("secondary epileptogenesis" in humans has remained controversial; see the chapter on medial temporal lobe epilepsy).

New Biomarkers of Epilepsy

A new marker of epilepsy beyond seizures and IEDs consists of the HFOs[3]. Two types of HFO are usually distinguished: ripples (120–250 Hz) and fast ripples (250–500 Hz). An important issue that has not yet been fully resolved in intracerebral EEG studies is the differentiation between normal HFOs related to cognitive activity and pathological HFOs related to epilepsy, which may occur in overlapping frequency ranges. In terms of amplitude, duration, and frequency, there exists a large overlap between physiological and pathological ripples found in normal and in epileptic conditions. Nonetheless, according to Gotman and Crone (2017), from the studies of HFOs recorded with intracranial EEG macroelectrodes, one can conclude that HFOs are important markers of the epileptogenic region not only in mesial temporal structures, where they are particularly abundant, but also in neocortical regions. Accordingly HFOs may be used as *biomarkers* of the epileptogenic zone. It should be noted that ripples (80–250 Hz) also occur in physiological conditions during memory consolidation processes in medial temporal structures, as shown by Jacobs et al. (2016). This same study reported also on the relation between the occurrence of HFOs and memory functions, suggesting that these oscillations may reflect a pathological process preventing normal memory functions. Several studies have shown the preferential activation of fast ripples during SWS (Staba et al., 2004). Another important feature of the SWS-related activation of local HFOs is their timely relation (coupling) to the up and down states of slow (<1 Hz) oscillations (Frauscher et al., 2015). This activation is apparently most intense in and around the seizure-initiating zone. This will be of utmost importance to better understand the relationship of epilepsy and plastic processes.

---

[3] HFO as a surrogate marker of epilepsy: To detect HFOs three technical requirements need to be fulfilled: (1) The usual sampling rate of the present commercial EEG machines is ca. 200 Hz (<500 Hz), enabling one to record from DC to 100 Hz. To record expanded bandwidth up to 600 Hz, 1–10 kHz is needed. The minimum acceptable sampling rate is 2.5 times greater than the highest frequency of interest. (2) Intracranial macroelectrodes: Commercial strip/grid, foramen ovale, and macro deep electrodes allow one to pick up ripples (R) and a certain amount of fast ripples (FR). Intracranial microwires are able to detect a wide range of HFOs (R + FR). (3) Differential and pass filters are needed to evaluate specific HFO activities. Several publications have demonstrated the possibility of detecting HFO activity through scalp leads.

THE RELATIONSHIP BETWEEN NON–RAPID EYE MOVEMENT SLEEP AND EPILEPTIC EVENTS AND THE UNDERLYING PHYSIOLOGIC MECHANISMS

The different types of epilepsies have complex interrelationships with sleep. Several excellent review papers have focused on this issue (Dinner and Lüders, 2001; Méndez and Radtke, 2001; Bazil, 2002; Foldvary-Schaefer and Grigg-Damberger, 2006).

The bond between sleep and epilepsy is presented in textbooks and clinical reviews mainly at the phenomenological level. This knowledge is summarized in the following tables.

Table 1.2 shows the occurrence of IEDs across vigilance states. It is clear that the major part emerges during SWS.

Table 1.3 demonstrates seizure proneness (across vigilance states) in different types of epilepsies. Both Tables 1.2 and 1.3 reveal that REM sleep may activate epileptic phenomena just in epilepsies involving limbic-temporal structures (but in the majority it does not); in addition SWS has an important activation potential in all types.

Table 1.4 shows both interictal and ictal sleep activation in different epilepsy syndromes. All epileptic manifestations and most epilepsies occur almost exclusively during SWS.

Table 1.5 highlights those specific patterns and situations clarified only by sleep studies.

TABLE 1.2   Propensity for Displaying Different Types of Interictal Epileptiform Discharges in Vigilance States

	Awake	NREM	REM	Trans
TLE spike	+	++	+	
ETLE spike	+	+	+	
SWD	++	++		++
ABS-like SW	+			+
GPFA		++		
Supr-burst	+	++		
ESES		+++		

ABS, absence; *ESES*, electrical status epilepticus in sleep; *ETLE*, extratemporal lobe epilepsy; *GPFA*, generalized paroxysmal fast activity; *NREM*, non–rapid eye movement; *REM*, rapid eye movement; *Supr-burst*, suppression-burst discharges; *SW*, spike–wave pattern; *SWD*, generalized spike–wave discharge; *TLE*, temporal lobe epilepsy; *Trans*, transitional states between awake–NREM and REM.

TABLE 1.3   Influence of Vigilance State on Syndrome-Dependent Interictal Epileptiform Discharges

	A S	A IED	NREM S	NREM IED	REM S	REM IED
IGE/absence	++	++	+++ (1–2 st)	+++	–	–
IGE/AW GTC	++ (Around awakening	+	–	+	–	–
IGE/JME	++ (Morning)	–+	–	+++ (Around awakening	–	–
MTLE	++ (GTC < CP)	+	++ (GTC > CP)	+++	+	+
NFLE	–	–	+++	+–	–	–
PE	+	+	+	++	+	+
BFCE	–	+	++	+++	–	+
LKS/ESES	–	++	–	++++	–	+
LGS	++	++	+++	++++	–	–
West	++ (Around awakening)	++	++	+++	+	+

A, awake; *AW GTC*, awakening generalized tonic–clonic seizures; *BFCE*, benign focal childhood epilepsies; *CP*, complex partial seizure; *GTC*, generalized tonic–clonic seizure; *IED*, interictal epileptiform discharge; *IGE*, idiopathic generalized epilepsy; *JME*, juvenile generalized myoclonic epilepsy; *LGS*, Lennox–Gastaut syndrome; *LKS/ESES*, Landau–Kleffner syndrome/electrical status epilepticus in sleep; *MTLE*, medial temporal lobe epilepsy; *NFLE*, nocturnal frontal lobe epilepsy; *NREM*, non–rapid eye movement; *PE*, partial epilepsy; *REM*, rapid eye movement; *S*, sleep; *st*, stage; *West*, West syndrome.

In this book, we try to grasp the neurophysiologic underpinnings of how NREM sleep activates epileptic manifestations. We aim at showing how this activation interferes with the plastic functions of sleep in several epileptic syndromes, causing chronic cognitive impairment.

Clinical and EEG symptoms of epilepsy preferentially manifest in relation to SWS. The occurrence of IEDs during SWS is not random; rather it may be linked either to CAP phase A1 (see the review by Parrino et al., 2000 and our results studying absence epilepsy in Chapter 2) or to sleep spindling (Terzano et al., 1991; Parrino et al., 2000; Beelke et al., 2000; Kellaway, 2000; Nobili et al., 2001). Spindles and slow waves are phenomena that are not so far from each other, both are parallel products of the corticothalamic system burst-firing mode during NREM sleep.

Újma et al. (2015) reported on the relationship between interictal cortical spikes captured by subdural electrodes and CAP A1 phase detected by scalp electrodes in epileptic patients under presurgical evaluation: spike activity was maximal during CAP A1 phase, suggesting a gating

TABLE 1.4   Influence of Vigilance State on Syndrome-Dependent Interictal Epileptiform Discharges and Seizures

	A S	A IED	NREM S	NREM IED	REM S	REM IED
IGE/ absence	++	–	+++ (1–2 st)	+++	–	–
IGE/AW GTC	++ (Around awakening	–	–	+	–	–
IGE/JME	++ (Morning)	–+	–	+++ (around awakening	–	–
MTLE	++ (GTC < CP)	+	+++ (GTC > CP)	+++	+	+
NFLE	–	–	+++	+–	–	–
PE	+	+	+	++	+	+
BFCE	–	+	++	+++	–	+
LKS/ESES	–	++	–	++++	–	+
LGS	++	++	+++	++++	–	–
West	++ (Around awakening)	++	++	+++	+	+

A, awake; AW GTC, awakening generalized tonic–clonic seizures; BFCE, benign focal childhood epilepsies; CP, complex partial seizure; IED, interictal epileptiform discharge; IGE, idiopathic generalized epilepsy; JME, juvenile generalized myoclonic epilepsy; LGS, Lennox–Gastaut syndrome; LKS/ESES, Landau–Kleffner syndrome/electrical status epilepticus in sleep; MTLE, medial temporal lobe epilepsy; NFLE, nocturnal frontal lobe epilepsy; NREM, non–rapid eye movement; PE, partial epilepsy; REM, rapid eye movement; S, sleep; st, stage; West, West syndrome.

TABLE 1.5   Strongly Sleep-Related EEG Patterns

Electrical status epilepticus in sleep (ESES)—exclusively during non–rapid eye movement (NREM) sleep

Generalized paroxysmal fast activity (GPFA) with polygraphic subtle ictal signs—almost always during NREM sleep

Generalized spike–wave bursts in the awakening generalized tonic–clonic form—almost exclusively during sleep in the awakening period

Focal sharps/spikes in frontal lobe epilepsies—frequently only during NREM sleep

Bilateral independent spiking in temporal lobe epilepsy—compared with wakefulness more frequently during NREM sleep

Centrotemporal uni- or bilateral spiking in rolandic epilepsy—compared to wakefulness more frequently in NREM sleep

In Lennox–Gastaut syndrome, to see both slow spike–waves (awake and in NREM sleep) and tonic miniseizures with GPFA in NREM sleep (stage 3)

Child with acquired aphasia and bilateral focal/secondary generalized perisylvian epileptiform activity to look for ESES function of slow waves. The association of CAP A1 phase with both interictal and ictal phenomena is noteworthy for two reasons: (1) It highlights that epileptiform phenomena are linked to sleep-like phasic shifts within the sleep microstructure. (2) The homeostatic sleep process regulates CAP A1 phase. Its prevalence increases with the augmentation of homeostatic pressure; therefore, epileptic activity is under the control of the same homeostatic process. Further studies may help to clarify these relations down to the neuronal membrane level regulating neuronal discharges.

Invasive presurgical investigations of epilepsy patients with subdural and deep electrodes may help in exploring the relation between cortical epileptiform potentials and different kinds of cortical oscillations. Frauscher et al. (2015) in Gotman's laboratory in Canada put in evidence the coupling of interictal discharges with slow ($<1\,Hz$) oscillations. Examining the gating effect of slow-wave up and down states on spike discharges, these authors found that spike and HFO density was highest during the transition from the up (depolarizing) state to the down (hyperpolarizing) state of the slow wave, a period of a high level of synchronization, unlike earlier ideas linking spike peaks to up states. Thus this activation of epileptiform activity during NREM sleep is not a state-dependent phenomenon, it is rather associated with specific phases of the slow-wave dynamics in which synchronization is enhanced. These authors interpreted this result as an argument supporting the conclusion that epileptiform phenomena (spike occurrence) are more associated with synchronization than with excitation. This rather unexpected finding may be accounted for by the fact that synchronization in the brain is mainly mediated by GABA A inhibitory mechanisms, mediated by GABA A receptor activation, which can facilitate the occurrence of spikes and HFOs (Avoli and de Curtis, 2011).

The strong cholinergic innervation and the related EEG desynchronization during REM sleep inhibit epileptiform discharges. Frauscher et al. (2016) investigated this link using scalp and intracerebral electrodes, discriminating tonic and phasic (with eye movements) REM phases. They found a stronger suppression of discharges during phasic than during tonic REM states. Ripples behaved differently in the spiking and nonspiking brain zones: HFOs increased during phasic REM in the normal (nonspiking) regions, whereas these increased during tonic REM in the spiking zones. This observation may have diagnostic value in the discrimination between pathological (epileptic; fast ripples) and physiological (cognitive) ripples (and regions) in the future. We may hypothesize that chronic cognitive impairments in epileptic patients are not the direct consequences of epileptic seizures and interictal discharges on brain functions, but result from the interference of IEDs and fast ripples with plastic sleep functions during NREM sleep. This possibility will be detailed throughout the further chapters of this book.

SOME MORE WORDS ABOUT OUR FRAME OF APPROACH

In this book, we will consider different epilepsy syndromes in an unorthodox way. These syndromes are introduced as network epilepsies linked to certain general physiological systems of the brain.

The network and system epilepsy concept goes beyond the now untenable focal/generalized dichotomy. According to this concept epileptic networks are linked to certain physiological brain systems/functions, which, on the one hand, may modulate epileptiform manifestations and, on the other, may be invaded and disrupted by the epileptic disorder. This may be most dramatic in the early phase of brain development, as seen in some epileptic syndromes. The conditions considered earlier to be "generalized" epilepsies may originate from specific networks very quickly, driving epileptic discharges bilaterally through the corticothalamic system; "focal" epilepsies are not strictly bound to a circumscribed region either, rather the epileptic activity can involve more or less widespread networks, sometimes in bilateral homologous regions (as in occipital and temporal lobe epilepsies).

Here we reinterpret several syndromes within the frameworks of system epilepsies. To give two examples: we introduce absence epilepsy as a system epilepsy linked to the sleep-promoting system activated by the shift from the awake state to NREM sleep, and autosome dominant nocturnal frontal lobe epilepsy as a system epilepsy of the arousal system, activated by (micro)arousals from sleep.

These two twin epilepsies "hijack" reciprocal antagonistic functions of the sleep/arousal system congruent with NREM sleep dynamics characterized by continuous up–down state oscillations of the sleep-promoting and the arousal systems (Halász, 2015; Halász, Bódizs, 2013).

Furthermore, we interpret medial temporal lobe epilepsy as the epilepsy of the declarative memory system, in view of the interference of hippocampal/temporal spiking with hippocampofrontal memory consolidation (Buzsáki, 2015), whereby electrophysiological actors of the memory function transform into exaggerated epileptic spiking and fast ripples.

We introduce benign regional childhood epilepsies with their malignant variants, electrical status epilepticus in sleep (ESES) and Landau–Kleffner syndrome (LKS), as the system epilepsies of the perisylvian cognitive network with severe regional (LKS) or diffuse cortical (ESES) involvement during sleep.

Our last examples of sleep-related system epilepsies are the epileptic encephalopathies (early epileptic encephalopathies, West syndrome, and Lennox–Gastaut syndrome), with abundant interictal and ictal epilepsy activation during NREM sleep.

Altogether, these sleep-related system epilepsies make up an important proportion of both childhood and adult epilepsies.

References

Achermann, P., Werth, E., Dijk, D.J., Borbely, A.A., 1995. Time course of sleep inertia after night time and daytime sleep episodes. Arch. Ital. Biol. 134 (1), 109–119.

Achermann, P., Finelli, L.A., Borbély, A.A., September 21 2001. Unihemispheric enhancement of delta power in human frontal sleep EEG by prolonged wakefulness. Brain Res. 913 (2), 220–223.

Aghakhani, Y., Bagshaw, A.P., Bénar, C.G., Hawco, C., Andermann, F., Dubeau, F., Gotman, J., 2004. FMRI activation during spike and wave discharges in idiopathic generalized epilepsy. Brain 27 (Pt. 5), 1127–1144.

Aghakhani, Y., Kobayashi, E., Bagshaw, A.P., Hawco, C., Bénar, C.G., Dubeau, F., Gotman, J., 2006. Cortical and thalamic fMRI responses in partial epilepsy with focal and bilateral synchronous spikes. Clin. Neurophysiol. 117 (1), 177–191.

Avanzini, G., Manganotti, P., Meletti, S., Moshé, S.L., Panzica, F., Wolf, P., Capovilla, G., 2012. The system epilepsies: a pathophysiological hypothesis. Epilepsia 53 (5), 771–778.

Avoli, M., de Curtis, M., 2011. GABA-ergic synchronization in the limbic system and its role in the generation of epileptiform activity. Progr, Neurobiol. 95, 104–132.

Bastien, C.H., Crowley, K.E., Colrain, I.M., 2002. Evoked potential components unique to non-REM sleep: relationship to evoked K-complexes and vertex sharp waves. Int. J. Psychophysiol. 46 (3), 257–274.

Bazil, C.W., 2002. Sleep and epilepsy. Semin. Neurol. 22 (3), 321–327.

Beenhakker, M.P., Huguenard, J.R., 2009. Neurons that fire together also conspire together: is normal sleep circuitry hijacked to generate epilepsy? Neuron 62 (5), 612–632.

Bellesi, M., Riedner, B.A., Garcia-Molina, G.N., Cirelli, C., Tononi, G., 2014. Enhancement of sleep slow waves: underlying mechanisms and practical consequences. Front. Syst. Neurosci. 28 (8), 208.

Beelke, M., Nobili, L., Baglietto, M.G., De Carli, F., Robert, A., De Negri, E., Ferrillo, F., 2000. Relationship of sigma activity to sleep interictal epileptic discharges: a study in children affected by benign epilepsy with occipital paroxysms. Epilepsy Res. 40 (2–3), 179–186.

Blume, W.T., 2001. Pathogenesis of Lennox-Gastaut syndrome: considerations and hypotheses. Epileptic Disord. 3 (4), 183–196.

Borbély, A.A., 1982. A two process model of sleep regulation. Hum. Neurobiol. 1 (3), 195–204.

Borbély, A.A., Baumann, F., Brandeis, D., Strauch, I., Lehmann, D., 1981. Sleep deprivation: effect on sleep stages and EEG power density in man. Electroencephalogr. Clin. Neurophysiol. 51 (5), 483–495.

Buzsáki, G., 29 1986. Hippocampal sharp waves: their origin and significance. Brain Res. 398 (2), 242–252.

Buzsáki, G., 2015. Hippocampal sharp wave-ripple: a cognitive biomarker for episodic memory and planning. Hippocampus 25 (10), 1073–1188.

Cajochen, C., Foy, R., Dijk, D.J., 1999. Frontal predominance of a relative increase in sleep delta and theta EEG activity after sleep loss in humans. Sleep Res. Online 2 (3), 65–69.

Capovilla, G., Moshé, S.L., Wolf, P., Avanzini, G., 2013. Epileptic encephalopathy as models of system epilepsy. Epilepsia 54 (Suppl. 8), 34–37.

Cash, S.S., Halgren, E., Dehghani, N., Rossetti, A.O., Thesen, T., Wang, C., Devinsky, O., Kuzniecky, R., Doyle, W., Madsen, J.R., Bromfield, E., Eross, L., Halász, P., Karmos, G., Csercsa, R., Wittner, L., Ulbert, I., May 22, 2009. The human K-complex represents an isolated cortical down-state. Science 324 (5930), 1084–1087.

Chugani, H.T., Shewmon, D.A., Sankar, R., Chen, B.C., Phelps, M.E., 1992. Infantile spasms: II. Lenticular nuclei and brain stem activation on positron emission tomography. Ann. Neurol. 31 (2), 212–219.

Colrain, I.M., 2005. The K-complex: a 7-decade history. Sleep 28 (2), 255–273.

Diagnostic Classification Steering Committee, Thorpy, M.J., 1990. International Classification of Sleep Disorders: Diagnostic and Coding Manual. American Sleep Disorders Association, Rochester, MN.

Dijk, D.J., Beersma, D.G., Daan, S., Bloem, G.M., Van den Hoofdakker, R.H., 1987. Quantitative analysis of the effects of slow wave sleep deprivation during the first 3 h of sleep on subsequent EEG power density. Eur. Arch. Psychiatry Neurol. Sci. 236 (6), 323–328.

Dinner, D.S., Lüders, H.O. (Eds.), 2001. Epilepsy and Sleep. Physiological and Clinical Relationships. Elsevier.

Fahoum, F., Lopes, R., Pittau, F., Dubeau, F., Gotman, J., 2012. Widespread epileptic networks in focal epilepsies: EEG-fMRI study. Epilepsia 53 (9), 1618–1627.

Finelli, L.A., Borbély, A.A., Achermann, P., 2001. Functional topography of the human non-REM sleep electroencephalogram. Eur. J. Neurosci. 13 (12), 2282–2290.

Foldvary-Schaefer, N., Grigg-Damberger, M., 2006. Sleep and epilepsy: what we know, don't know, and need to know. J. Clin. Neurophysiol. 23 (1), 4–20.

Frauscher, B., von Ellenrieder, N., Ferrari-Marinho, T., Avoli, M., Dubeau, F., et al., 2015. Facilitation of epileptic activity during sleep is mediated by high amplitude slow waves. Brain 138 (Pt. 6).

Frauscher, B., von Ellenrieder, N., Dubeau, F., Gotman, J., 2016. EEG desynchronization during phasic REM sleep suppresses interictal epileptic activity in humans. Epilepsia 57 (6), 879–888.

Goddard, G.V., 1983. The kindling model of epilepsy. Trends Neurosci. 6 (7), 275–279.

Gorter, A.J., van Vliet, E.A., Lopes da Silva, 2016. Which insights have we gained from the kindling and post-status epilepticus models. J. Neurosci. Methods 260 (SI), 96–108.

Gotman, J., Grova, C., Bagshaw, A., Kobayashi, E., Aghakhani, Y., Dubeau, F., 2005. Generalized epileptic discharges show thalamocortical activation and suspension of the default state of the brain. Proc. Natl. Acad. Sci. U. S. A. 102 (42), 15236–15240.

Gotman, J., Crone, N.E., 2017. High frequency oscillation. In: Schomer, D.L., Lopes da Silva, F.H. (Eds.), Niedermexer's Electroencephalography. Oxford University Press, New York, pp. 749–766.

Haegelen, C., Perucca, P., Châtillon, C.E., Andrade-Valença, L., Zelmann, R., Jacobs, J., Collins, D.L., Dubeau, F., Olivier, A., Gotman, J., 2013. High-frequency oscillations, extent of surgical resection, and surgical outcome in drug-resistant focal epilepsy. Epilepsia 54 (5), 848–857.

Halász, P., Kundra, O., Rajna, P., Pál, I., Vargha, M., 1979. Micro-arousals during nocturnal sleep. Acta Physiol. Acad. Sci. Hung 54 (1), 1–12.

Halász, P., 2005. K-complex, a reactive EEG graphoelement of NREM sleep: an old chap in a new garment. Sleep Med. Rev. 9, 391–412.

Halász, P., Bódizs, R., 2013. Dynamic Structure of NREM Sleep. Sringer, London.

Halász, P., Bódizs, R., Parrino, L., Terzano, M., 2014. Two features of sleep slow waves: homeostatic and reactive aspects–from long term to instant sleep homeostasis. Sleep Med. 15 (10), 1184–1195.

Halász, P., 2015. Are absence epilepsy and nocturnal frontal lobe epilepsy system epilepsies of the sleep/wake system? Behav. Neurol. 2015. Article ID: 231676.

Horne, J.A., Wilkinson, S., 1985. Chronic sleep reduction: daytime vigilance performance and EEG measures of sleepiness, with particular reference to "practice" effects. Psychophysiology 22 (1), 69–78.

Höller, Y., Kutil, R., Klaffenböck, L., Thomschewski, A., Höller, P.M., Bathke, A.C., Jacobs, J., Taylor, A.C., Nardone, R., Trinka, E., 2015. HFO in epilepsy and surgical outcome. A meta-analysis. Front. Humman Neurosci. 20 (9), 574.

Huber, R., Ghilardi, M.F., Massimini, M., Ferrarelli, F., Riedner, B.A., Peterson, M.J., Tononi, G., 2006. Arm immobilization causes cortical plastic changes and locally decreases sleep slow wave activity. Nat. Neurosci. 9 (9), 1169–1176.

Jacobs, J., Vogt, C., LeVan, P., Zelmann, R., Gotman, J., Kobayashi, K., 2016. The identification of distinct high-frequency oscillations during spikes delineates the seizure onset zone better than high-frequency spectral power changes. Clin. Neurophysiol. 127 (1), 129–142.

Jacobs, J., Zijlmans, M., Zelmann, R., Chatillon, C.E., Hall, J., Olivier, A., Dubeau, F., Gotman, J., 2010. High-frequency electroencephalographic oscillations correlate with outcome of epilepsy surgery. Ann. Neurol. 67 (2), 209–220.

Jefferys, G.J., Menendez de la Prida, Wendling, F., Bragin, A., Avoli, M., Timofeev, I., Lopes da Silva, F.H., 2012. Mechanisms of physiological and epileptic HFO generation. Progr. Neurobiol. 98 (3), 250–264.

Jensen, F.E., 2011. Epilepsy as a spectrum disorder: implications from novel clinical and basic neuroscience. Epilepsia 52 (Suppl. 1), 1–6.

Kattler, H., Dijk, D.J., Borbély, A.A., 1994. Effect of unilateral somatosensory stimulation prior to sleep on the sleep EEG in humans. J. Sleep Res. 3 (3), 159–164.

Kellaway, P., 2000. The electroencephalographic features of benign centrotemporal (rolandic) epilepsy of childhood. Epilepsia 41 (8), 1053–1056.

Krueger, J.M., Obál, F., 1993. A neuronal group theory of sleep function. J. Sleep Res. 2 (2), 63–69.

Laurino, M., Menicucci, D., Piarulli, A., Mastorci, F., Bedini, R., Allegrini, P., Gemignani, A., 2014. Disentangling different functional roles of evoked K-complex components: mapping the sleeping brain while quench hing sensory processing. Neuroimage 86, 433–445.

Loomis, A.L., Harvey, E.N., Hobart, G.A., 1937. Cerebral states during sleep as studies by human brain potentials. J. Exp. Psychol. 21, 127–144.

Lüders, H.O., Awad, I., 1992. Conceptual considerations. In: Lüders, H.O. (Ed.), Epilepsy Surgery. Raven Press, New York, pp. 51–62.

Marzano, C., Ferrara, M., Curcio, G., De Gennaro, L., 2010. The effects of sleep deprivation in humans: topographical electroencephalogram changes in non-rapid eye movement (NREM) sleep versus REM sleep. J. Sleep Res. 19 (2), 260–268.

Massimini, M., Ferrarelli, F., Esser, S.K., Riedner, B.A., Huber, R., et al., 2007. Triggering sleep slow waves by transcranial magnetic stimulation. Proc. Natl. Acad. Sci. U. S. A. 104 (20), 8496–8501.

Meletti, S., Ruggieri, A., Avanzini, P., Caramaschi, E., Filippini, M., Bergonzini, P., Monti, G., Vignoli, A., Olivotto, S., Mastrangelo, M., Santucci, M., Gobbi, G., Veggiotti, P., Vaudano, A.E., 2016. Extrastriate visual cortex in idiopathic occipital epilepsies: the contribution of retinotopic areas to spike generation. Epilepsia 57 (6), 896–906.

Méndez, M., Radtke, R.A., 2001. Interactions between sleep and epilepsy. J. Clin. Neurophysiol. 18 (2), 106–127.

Mesulam, M.M., 1998. From sensation to cognition. Brain. 121 (Pt. 6), 1013–1052. http://www.ncbi.nlm.nih.gov/pubmed/9648540.

Navlakha, S., Barth, A.L., Bar-Joseph, Z., 2015. Decreasing-rate pruning optimizes the construction of efficient and robust distributed networks. PLoS Comput. Biol. 11 (7).

Ngo, H.V., Claussen, J.C., Born, J., Mölle, M., 2013. Induction of slow oscillations by rhythmic acoustic stimulation. J. Sleep Res. 22 (1), 22–31.

Nobili, L., Baglietto, M.G., Beelke, M., De Carli, F., De Negri, E., Gaggero, R., Rosadini, G., Veneselli, E., Ferrillo, F., 2001. Distribution of epileptiform discharges during nREM sleep in the CSWSS syndrome: relationship with sigma and delta activities. Epilepsy Res. 44 (2–3), 119–128.

Parrino, L., Smerieri, A., Spaggiari, M.C., Terzano, M.G., 2000. Cyclic alternating pattern (CAP) and epilepsy during sleep: how a physiological rhythm modulates a pathological event. Clin. Neurophysiol. 111 (Suppl. 2), S39–S46.

Pittau, F., Grova, C., Moeller, F., Dubeau, F., Gotman, J., 2012. Patterns of altered functional connectivity in mesial temporal lobe epilepsy. Epilepsia 53 (6), 1013–1023.

Rechtschaffen, A., Kales, A., 1968. A Manual of Standardized Terminology, Techniques and Scoring System for Sleep Stages of Human Subjects. University of California, Brain Information Service/Brain Research Institute, Los Angeles, CA.

Riedner, B.A., Hulse, B.K., Murphy, M.J., Ferrarelli, F., Tononi, G., 2011. Temporal dynamics of cortical sources underlying spontaneous and peripherally evoked slow waves. Progr. Brain Res. 193, 201–218.

Rosenow, F., Lüders, H., 2001. Presurgical evaluation of epilepsy. Brain 124 (Pt. 9), 1683–1700.

Schieber, J.P., Muzet, A., Ferierre, P.J.R., 1971. Les phases d'activation transitoire spontanées su cours du sommeil normal chez l'homme. Arch. Sci. Physiol. 25, 443–465.

Spencer, S.S., 2002. Neural networks in human epilepsy: evidence of and implications for treatment. Epilepsia 43 (3), 219–227.

Stahnisch, F.W., Nitsch, R., November 2002. Santiago Ramón y Cajal's concept of neuronal plasticity: the ambiguity lives on. Trends Neurosci. 25 (11), 589–591.

Staba, R.J., Wilson, C.L., Bragin, A., Jhung, D., Fried, I., Engel Jr., J., 2004. High-frequency oscillations recorded in human medial temporal lobe during sleep. Ann. Neurol. 56 (1), 108–115.

Steriade, M., 2003. Neuronal Substrates of Sleep and Epilepsy. Cambridge University Press, pp. 322–370.

Takahashi, K., Kayama, Y., Lin, J.S., Sakai, K., 2010. Locus coeruleus neuronal activity during the sleep-waking cycle in mice. Neuroscience 169 (3), 1115–1126.

Terzano, M.G., Mancia, D., Salati, M.R., Costani, G., Decembrino, A., et al., 1985. The cyclic alternating pattern as a physiologic component of normal NREM sleep. Sleep 8 (2), 13.

Terzano, M.G., Parrino, L., Boselli, M., Smerieri, A., Spaggiari, M.C., 2000. CAP components and EEG synchronization in the first 3 sleep cycles. Clin. Neurophysiol. 111 (2), 283–290.

Terzano, M.G., Parrino, L., Spaggiari, M.C., Barusi, R., Simeoni, S., 1991. Discriminatory effect of cyclic alternating pattern in focal lesional and benign rolandic interictal spikes during sleep. Epilepsia 32 (5), 616–628.

Tononi, G., Cirelli, C., 2003. Sleep and synaptic homeostasis: a hypothesis. Brain Res. Bull. 62 (2), 143–150.

Tseng, S.H., Tsai, L.Y., Yeh, S.R., 9 2008. Induction of high-frequency oscillations in a junction-coupled network. J. Neurosci. 28 (28), 7165–7173.

Ujszászi, J., Halász, P., 1988. Long latency evoked potential components in human slow wave sleep. Electroencephalogr. Clin. Neurophysiol. 69 (6), 516–522.

Vyazovskiy, V., Borbély, A.A., Tobler, I., 2000. Unilateral vibrissae stimulation during waking induces interhemispheric EEG asymmetry during subsequent sleep in the rat. J. Sleep Res. 9 (4), 367–371.

Vyazovskiy, V.V., Faraguna, U., Cirelli, C., Tononi, G., 2009. Triggering slow waves during NREM sleep in the rat by intracortical electrical stimulation: effects of sleep/wake history and background activity. J. Neurophysiol. 101 (4), 1921–1931.

Wolf, P., Yacubian, E.M., Avanzini, G., Sander, T., Schmitz, B., Wandschneider, B., Koepp, M., 2015. Juvenile myoclonic epilepsy: a system disorder of the brain. Epilepsy Res. 114, 2–12.

Wolf, P., 2015. Reflex epileptic mechanisms in humans: lessons about natural ictogenesis. Epilepsy Behav. 52 (Pt. A), 277–278.

Absence Epilepsy as the System Epilepsy of the Non–Rapid Eye Movement Sleep-Promoting System

ABSENCE EPILEPSY AS THE SYSTEM EPILEPSY OF THE NON–RAPID EYE MOVEMENT SLEEP-PROMOTING SYSTEM

Absences are frequent epileptic manifestations of childhood and young adulthood, characterized by ~3-Hz bilateral spike-and-wave discharges (SWDs) on the EEG. Absences make up the only seizure type of childhood absence epilepsy, appearing also in other idiopathic epilepsy syndromes like juvenile absence epilepsy, juvenile myoclonic epilepsy (JME), and eyelid myoclonia with absences (Jeavons syndrome). Although the pheno- and genotypes of these epilepsy syndromes are different, they share electroclinical symptoms, i.e., absences, and a common pathomechanism.

In the following sections, the possible links of absences and SWDs with sleep will be analyzed:

1. the relation of absences with sleep-promoting brain mechanisms (shown by certain sleep EEG elements)
2. the timing of absences across the wake/sleep process
3. the effect of phasic sensory input on the occurrence of absence seizures on different levels of homeostatic pressure and vigilance
4. what is common and what is different between the neurophysiology of absences/SWDs and slow-wave sleep

THE RELATIONSHIP OF THE CORTICOTHALAMIC SYSTEM AND ABSENCE SEIZURES WITH BILATERAL SYNCHRONOUS SPIKE–WAVE DISCHARGES

The thalamus (Williams, 1965; Jasper and Droogleever-Fortuyn, 1974) has long been linked to the pathomechanism of absences and SWD. Pierre Gloor (1968), from the Montreal Neurological Institute, was a pioneer in calling attention to the role of the corticothalamic (called by him "corticoreticular") system and the sleep system after a long and fruitless debate on the cortical/subcortical origin of SWDs.

THE TWO WORKING MODES OF THE CORTICOTHALAMIC SYSTEM IN WAKING AND NON–RAPID EYE MOVEMENT SLEEP

The Transformation of the Sleep Working Mode to the Bilateral Spike–Wave Pattern

The system works as a relay center during wakefulness, faithfully conveying the input from the outside world toward the cortex. This is realized by the "tonic activity" of the network reflected by a desynchronized EEG. The EEG desynchronized activity/tonic mode is transformed during non–rapid eye movement (NREM) sleep to a synchronized rhythmic EEG activity: slow waves and spindles. This is the "burst-firing" working mode interrupting the information flow from the outside world to the cortex (Steriade, 2003a). Its cellular substrate mainly relates to special membrane and receptor characteristics of the participating cells and their wiring (McCromick and Bal, 1997; Huguenard and McCormick, 2007). The membrane conductance of thalamic neurons is characterized by the presence of a low-threshold T-type Ca^{2+} channel, which, during their bursting-mode activity, amplifies the thalamic oscillations. In the waking state, the T current is inactive, not interfering with the transmission of stimuli. The waking state is maintained by the effect of the ascending brain stem activating system. When we go to sleep, a cascade of events occurs changing the working mode of the thalamocortical system. The de-inactivation of the low-threshold Ca^{2+} current dominates the functional profile of the thalamic neurons in their hyperpolarized state compared to the resting membrane potentials in waking. This transition occurs during drowsiness and on the borderlands from waking to slow-wave sleep, while the ascending arousal decreases. Under such conditions the relay neurons respond, with a rebound Ca^{2+} burst, to the inhibitory feedback coming from the thalamic reticular nucleus (RE). Because the RE innervates large thalamic neuronal populations, synchronized GABAergic (both GABA A and GABA B) inhibitory postsynaptic potentials de-inactivate low-threshold Ca^{2+} current spikes in a number of thalamic neurons, initiating rebound excitation. The low-threshold Ca^{2+} current spikes correspond to the spindle waves. This excitation then reactivates the RE and activates the cortex. The reactivated RE initiates an inhibitory postsynaptic potential in the thalamic neurons forming a second spindle wave. The hyperpolarization of the thalamic neurons reopens the way for the activation of spike bursts based on Ca^{2+}

current, and the whole excitatory–inhibitory cycle involving the RE and thalamic relay cells is set into motion again. The RE is the driving force of spindling (Steriade et al., 1985). Thalamic structures isolated from the RE do not show oscillatory behavior, but even an isolated RE produces spindling. NREM sleep is induced by the inhibitory influences originating from the basal forebrain on brain stem arousal centers, releasing the thalamocortical system from the inhibition coming from the ascending reticular arousal system.

From Bursting Mode to Spike–Wave Pattern

After the exploration of the phasic inhibitory gating exerted by the RE on the thalamocortical circuit, it has become clear that this mechanism could be the basis of the spike–wave pattern in absence epilepsy. Gloor et al. (1990) assumed that the same thalamic volley eliciting spindles on the cortex in normal sleep evokes the spike–wave pattern. This was seen in the experiment of Kostopoulos et al. (1981), who applied intramuscular penicillin to cats, increasing the cortical excitability (Fig. 2.1). They also showed that the arousal influences could block spike–wave paroxysms by depolarizing the thalamic relay cells; whereas shifts toward sleep promoted their appearance. The possible role of the increased function of low-threshold Ca^{2+} current in the thalamic (RE and relay cell) neurons has become more and more evident. This would classify idiopathic generalized epilepsies (IGEs)

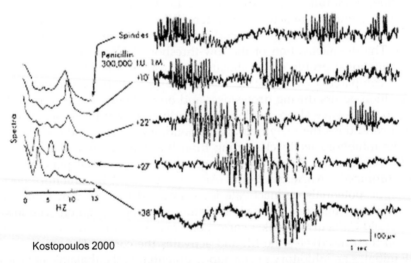

FIGURE 2.1   Kostopoulos's (1981) experimental work with penicillin, a GABA-inhibitory substance. Penicillin injected intramuscularly (*IM*) into cats transforms sleep spindling to spike–wave discharges. Numbers indicate the time elapsed from the injection.

in the group of channelopathies. A different concept was given by Bal et al. (1995a,b) and others (Huguenard and Prince, 1994; Sanchez-Vives et al., 1995). The pharmacological blockage of GABA A receptors in ferret geniculate slices resulted in the transformation of spindle waves into paroxysmal activity, so that both the thalamocortical and the perigeniculate neurons greatly increased the intensity of their burst discharges and became phase locked into a 2- to 4-Hz rhythm. This phenomenon suggested that this shift from normal to paroxysmal activity could result from the disinhibition of perigeniculate neurons from one another, leading to an increase in the discharge rate of these cells and a large increase in the postsynaptic activation of GABA B receptors in the thalamocortical neurons. Thus, the spindle waves slowly transformed into a paroxysmal oscillation that resembled a spike-and-wave pattern. However, the thalamocortical circuit may be influenced via several ascending and descending pathways from the brain stem and the cortex. Therefore, it is not surprising that the same distortion of functions resulting in epileptic SWDs in the system could stem from influences of different key points in the network. Pharmacological factors in play external to the thalamocortical circuitry include cholinergic, dopaminergic, noradrenergic, and serotoninergic mechanisms. Pathways that utilize these various transmitters project onto the thalamus and/or cortex from sites distant to those structures and may modulate the process from the top or the bottom. Perturbation in one or more of these neuronal networks may lead to abnormal neuronal oscillatory rhythms within the thalamocortical system, with a consequent generation of bilaterally synchronous SWDs featuring IGE.

The Montreal school (Gloor and Fariello, 1988) emphasized the coexistence of three components that may promote the development of IGE-like epileptic states: increased excitability of the cortex, weakness of the brain stem tonic arousal influence, and the phasically inhibited thalamocortical stream of impulses, now known as the "bursting mode" of the thalamocortical system.

Gloor (1968) proposed that SWDs, the EEG substrate of absences, emerge from the same circuit that normally produces sleep spindles. The former are epileptic transformations of the latter. This idea fertilized further research, reaching out until now. In his later work, Kostopoulos (2000) provided further arguments supporting the spindle transformation theory.

Another important line of studies on the "cortical drivers" of the spike–wave pattern evolved in the last decade of the 19th century. Meeren et al. (2002, 2005), from the Nijmegen laboratory of experimental neurosciences, dealing long ago with the enigma of the spike–wave pattern of absence seizures, described cortical seizure onset spots in the genetic absence model of rats, entraining secondarily very quickly the frontal cortex and thalamic corticoreticular structures into a bilateral synchronous oscillation in the form of a spike–wave pattern. In later papers the several interesting molecular features of the driver zones were characterized (Manning et al., 2004; Klein et al., 2004), and a successful therapeutic approach has also been described (Blumenfeld et al., 2008). Avoli (2012), in a review paper, summarized the brief history of the oscillatory roles of the thalamus and cortex in absence seizures.

Almost in parallel Steriade (2003a,b,c) summarized contemporary results about sleep and epilepsy in his epoch-marking book. In his own work he showed on chronically implanted, freely moving, naturally awake and sleeping cats that in absence-like seizures SWDs "originate in the neocortex and are disseminated through mono-oligo and multi-synaptic intracortical circuits, before they spread to the thalamus and exhibit generalized features." The Steriade group has supported the cortical origin of absences with several ablation experiments. They also stressed the propagation dynamics of the seizures from focal to widespread, confirming early observations in humans, suggesting a focal onset (Bancaud et al., 1974; Niedermeyer et al., 1969, 1972).

New technical advances in human neurophysiological recordings demonstrate the possibility of searching for possible sources of spike–waves in absences in the human cortex using a dense array of multiple electrodes (Holmes et al., 2004). Also magnetoencephalography recordings in children (Westmijse et al., 2009; Tenney and Glauser, 2013) have evidenced the focal frontal onset of absences.

This is a complete breach with the old "centrencephalic" theory of Penfield (Jasper, 1977), who had hypothesized a midline deep (thalamic) source of SWDs. Nowadays we rather believe that the apparently bilaterally and synchronously appearing absences are initiated by unilateral frontal cortical zones entraining the frontal cortex and the nonspecific thalamic structures within some milliseconds.

Although it is clear now that there are no bilaterally projecting thalamic neurons, the influential centrencephalic theory and the associated "secondary bilateral synchrony" hypothesis of Tükel and Jasper (1952) have survived in several clinical papers. Although the cortical origin of SWDs is clear now, we still need to see the crucial role of the thalamus in shaping the special absence/spike–wave mechanism. During cortical seizures with 3-Hz spike–wave complexes, the cells of the RE produce a spike burst in line with inhibitory postsynaptic potentials of the thalamocortical (TC) neurons (Steriade, 2003a,b) (Figs. 2.2 and 2.3). Thus, the GABAergic RE neurons are actively involved in the circuit, generating SWDs and spindles. Concerning the "wave" component of the SWD Steriade was inclined to interpret it as "disfacilitation" and not a GABAergic inhibition, as a hyperpolarization phase of down states within the <1-Hz slow oscillation (Steriade, 2003c).

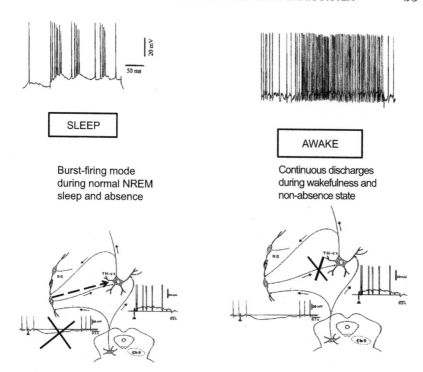

FIGURE 2.2   Two kinds of corticothalamic system working mode: continuous in waking and in seizure-free state (right side) and intermittent in non–rapid eye movement sleep and during epileptic absences (left side). Unit discharges in the cortex are continuous (right) or intermittent (=burst-firing) (left). The blood flow decreases and the cortical activity is deactivated (disfacilitated) in a mosaic-like pattern. The diagrams of the thalamocortical system (bottom right and left) show the liberated thalamic reticular nucleus (RE)–thalamic inhibition (*dashed black arrow*) related to the depression of the inhibitory influence on the RE reticular ascending system (*black cross*) during absences (left) and to the suspended RE–thalamic inhibition (*black cross*) during the waking and seizure-free state (right). *Ch S*, cholinergic neuron in the mesencephalic ascending arousal system providing the RE neurons with inhibitory innervation to the thalamocortical relay cells producing excitatory impulses; *fMR*, functional magnetic resonance; *RE*, thalamic reticular nucleus neuron; *SPECT*, single photon emission computerized tomography; *TCD*, transcranial Doppler; *TH-cx*, thalamo-cortical neuron.

Beenhakker and Huguenard (2009) dedicated their interesting paper to mechanisms by which epilepsy "hijacks" certain sleep-related circuits. They reinvestigated the relationship of sleep spindles and SWDs by contemporary neurophysiological methods. One of the prevailing views is that the blockade of GABA A receptors promotes the switch from spindling to SWDs (McCromick and Bal, 1997; Huguenard and McCormick, 2007) by eliminating intra-RE inhibition of normal sleep spindling.

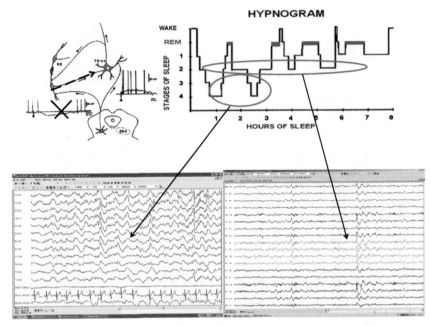

FIGURE 2.3   Top left: Steriade's schema of the corticothalamic system in burst-firing working mode during non–rapid eye movement (NREM) sleep (*Ch S*, cholinergic neuron in the mesencephalic ascending arousal system providing the RE neurons with inhibitory innervation to the thalamocortical relay cells producing excitatory impulses; *RE*, thalamic reticular nucleus neuron; *TH-cx*, thalamocortical neuron). During NREM sleep the inhibitory influence on RE neurons (*thick dashed arrow*) is liberated from the inhibitory influence of the brain stem reticular ascending system (*black cross*, placed on the inhibitory postsynaptic potential) (see also in Fig. 2.2). Bottom: EEGs of NREM sleep stages 2 (right) and 3 (left). The NREM sleep EEG is the product of the burst-firing mode working of the corticothalamic system. Top right: The conventional hypnogram showing the place of the second and third sleep stages in the sleep cycle.

Several gene mutations have been found to be involved in the genesis of absences; however, the relevant epileptogenic modifications in human absence epilepsy have not been identified. Whatever the mechanisms, there is a strong support for the thesis that normal thalamic functional circuits working during NREM sleep provide a template for epileptic circuits; in other words, normal sleep circuitry is hijacked by epilepsy.

For example, RE neurons contain the GABA A receptor β3 subunit, whereas those receptors expressed by the TC neurons do not. Genetically removing the β3 subunit from mice eliminates the intra-RE inhibition, but it does not affect RE-to-TC inhibition. β3-knockout mice have robust and synchronous thalamic oscillations (like in epilepsy); and these mice have an Angelman syndrome–like phenotype including absence-type seizures. Thus reducing intra-RE inhibition is likely to contribute to absences.

The electrical coupling among RE neurons might contribute to absences through the electrical coupling of RE neurons leading to a hypersynchrony of RE neurons during SWDs (Von Krosigk et al., 1993; Kim et al., 1997). Congruently, carbenoxelone, and inhibitor of gap-junctional communication, reduces the number and duration of SWDs in animal models of absence epilepsy (Deleuze and Huguenard, 2006).

Several factors may influence the RE neurons' excitability. The most potent absence- and spike–wave-promoting agent is the excitatory input originating from the cortex, able to transform the spindles to 3-Hz SWD oscillations. Ample variations may occur via the up- and downregulation of the excitatory/inhibitory balance in cortical, thalamic, and reticular neurons. Because the corticothalamic circuit is influenced via several ascending and descending pathways from the brain stem and the cortex, it is not surprising that the dysfunction resulting in epileptic SWDs may originate from different points in the network.

THE INFLUENCE OF VIGILANCE CHANGES ACROSS THE SLEEP–WAKE AND THE CIRCADIAN CYCLES ON THE RELEASE OF ABSENCES

A very close link between the level of vigilance and the expression of SWDs was recognized in the 1970s (Fig. 2.4). Early studies have proven that spontaneous paroxysms are promoted by transitory vigilance drops: after awakening in the morning, after lunch, during evening sleepiness, in boring situations (Slaght et al., 2002; Gareri et al., 2005; Passouant, 1971), and in experimental depression of the reticular arousal system (Stevens et al., 1971). Whole-night studies had similar results: 3-Hz generalized SWDs selectively occur in the transitional periods of NREM sleep, as well as in wakefulness and REM sleep (Janz, 1974; Gloor et al., 1973; Halász and Dévényi, 1974). In addition, animal studies have confirmed this tendency (Niedermeyer, 1967, 1972). The spike–wave pattern is absent during REM sleep in both humans and animals (Gloor, 1968; Drinkenburg et al., 1991); however, in those periods in which REM sleep is fragmented by elements of NREM sleep (sleep spindles and vertex sharp waves) or wakefulness (alpha spindles), SWDs may appear (Halász and Dévényi, 1974).

There are very few works aiming to clarify how absences distribute in relation to circadian rhythms. This approach requires a highly sophisticated experimental setup, because absence epilepsy is closely associated with vigilance level changes. Therefore, all studies looking for clock-time circadian seizure occurrence of absences without controlling the actual vigilance state have serious limitations confounding the two effects. Tomka (1985) registered 30 absence epilepsy patients

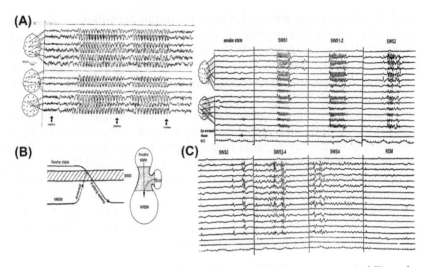

FIGURE 2.4   The vigilance dependency of absences. (A) Absences appear in falling asleep and are inhibited by arousing stimuli. (B) A critically decreased level of vigilance between somnolence and superficial sleep stage 2 promotes absences through oscillations especially by shifts toward sleep. (C) Absences appear on this level, even when they are absent in the previous waking state. They disappear in deeper sleep and are absent in rapid eye movement (REM) sleep. Nonictal variants of spike–wave activity, however, are present during the whole non–rapid eye movement (NREM) sleep. SWD, spike–wave discharge; SWS, slow-wave sleep.

with 37 all-night polygraph recordings. The preponderance of absences was the highest during "hypersynchronous alpha states" contrasting with full wakefulness. Smyk et al. (2011) investigated the spontaneous rhythm of seizure occurrence in the Wag/Rij rat model of absence epilepsy. They registered the motor activity, circadian parameters, SWDs, and sleep–wake states. SWDs typically preceded passive wakefulness and slow-wave sleep. The results suggested the independence of spike–wave generation from the circadian timing system. Zarowski et al. (2011) studied the circadian distribution and sleep–wake patterns of children's generalized seizures. Absence seizures occurred predominantly during wakefulness from 9:00 a.m. to noon and from 6:00 p.m. to midnight; the state of vigilance preceding the seizures was not analyzed.

Pavlova et al. (2009) measured in five generalized epilepsy patients (four with juvenile myoclonic type) the timing of interictal SWDs in relation with their hourly plasma melatonin level for evaluating circadian rhythmicity. Most SWDs occurred during NREM sleep (NREM/wake ratio 14:1). In the two patients who had NREM sleep in all circadian phases there was a clear circadian variation in SWDs but with different phases compared to the melatonin peaks. This pilot study supports the existence of a circadian modulation of discharges beyond the obvious NREM control (note that just short spike–wave paroxysms not fulfilling the criteria for the length of behavioral absences were analyzed in this study).

Based upon clinical observations, absences have been considered awake events. However, they occur during decreased levels of vigilance even when emerging within the waking domain and even in stage 1–2 sleep (Tomka, 1985; Smyk et al., 2011). Several studies have proven that absences are halted by arousing stimuli causing a sudden rise in vigilance (Rajna and Lona, 1989). The vigilance level dependency of absences explains their distribution throughout the 24-h sleep–wake cycle (Zarowski et al., 2011). An important proportion of seizures are hidden during light NREM sleep or around transitory phases to and from sleeping/wakefulness as well as to and from REM/NREM sleep. The preferential zones are not only periods with decreased vigilance, but also those with a high rate of vigilance oscillations between higher and deeper levels (Halász and Dévényi, 1974; Coenen et al., 1991).

CAN EXPERIMENTAL MANIPULATIONS OF THE HYPOTHALAMIC SLEEP-PROMOTING SYSTEM ELICIT ABSENCES?

Additional support was given for the strong link between absence epilepsy and the sleep system by the study of Suntsova et al. (2009) on Wag/Rij rats, a genetic absence strain. Absence-like seizures were elicited in the nonepileptic animals by fractional electrical stimulation of the sleep-promoting hypothalamic neurons.

SPIKE–WAVE DISCHARGES ELICITED BY SENSORY STIMULI AND LINKED TO THE SLOW-WAVE TYPE OF PHASIC EVENTS

Looking into the dynamic features of the peculiar transitional states of vigilance, a high amount of bidirectional oscillations between sleep and arousal can be found. Applying sensory stimulation for manipulating vigilance oscillations, we have shown that the majority of the "spontaneous" spike–wave paroxysms occur during fluctuations toward NREM sleep compared to fluctuations toward wakefulness or REM sleep (Halász et al., 2002,b). Sensory stimuli increased the vigilance fluctuations in line with the number of spike–wave paroxysms.

The sleep EEG analysis of 10 primary generalized epileptic patients performed by Terzano et al. (1989) after the recognition of the cyclic alternating pattern (CAP) phenomenon showed the preponderance of SWDs during CAP phases. The analysis of the sleep distribution of SWDs in 10 JME patients (Gigli et al., 1992) revealed that the spike rate was significantly higher in CAP A phase compared to non-CAP, and the spikes were strongly inhibited during the CAP B phase. These data confirmed prior results on the association of sleep level fluctuations with SWDs, and supported finding on the impact of shifts toward slow-wave sleep. The strong correlation between absences and reactive (evoked) sleep slow waves (Halász et al., 2002,b) is another strong argument supporting the link between absences and shifts toward NREM sleep.

In IGE patients, 70% of SWD occurred during CAP A1, 24% in A2, and 6% in A3 (Parrino et al., 2000). Consequently, the amount of SWDs was the highest in the first sleep cycles, declining later, paralleling the decay of the delta power from evening to morning (Fig. 2.5). The CAP-related activation of SWDs was threefold on the descending slopes dominated by subtypes A1 compared to the ascending slopes containing more A2 and A3 events.

Studying frontal and generalized SWDs in 13 children with absence epilepsy Koutroumanidis et al. (2012) found that the generalized discharges tended to occur during sleep fluctuations, especially when sleep shifted from the B to the A phase of CAP. Also this finding supports the notion, that the fine-graded shifts toward NREM sleep gate SWD.

There is growing evidence on the impact of the frontal lobe on NREM sleep slow oscillations, including CAP A phases (Ferri et al., 2008) and SWDs as well.

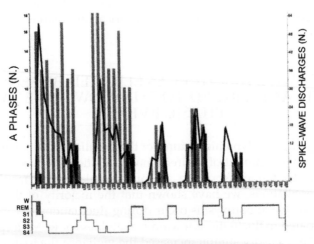

FIGURE 2.5   The distribution of absences across the sleep cycle. Absences prevail during the first two cycles and during the descending slopes of the cycles in which the homeostatic sleep pressure is the highest. *REM*, rapid eye movement; *S1*, non–rapid eye movement (NREM) sleep stage 1; *S2*, NREM sleep stage 2; *S3*, NREM stage 3; *S4*, NREM stage 4; *W*, wake.

The well-known activating effect of sleep deprivation might be related to the increased chance of clashes between sleep- and wakefulness-promoting forces, resulting in more vigilance fluctuations, with the outcome of more swings toward NREM sleep (Halász et al., 2002a,).

The apparent association of absences with arousal (Niedermeyer 1991) needs to be treated with caution, because even when they appear to be elicited by an arousal, a more elaborate analysis may reveal that such absences are actually linked to the reactive sleep-like antiarousal responses (Halász, 1982).

COMMON AND DIFFERENT NEUROPHYSIOLOGIC AND NEUROIMAGING FEATURES OF ABSENCES AND SLEEP

For further evaluation of the hypothesis that absence epilepsy associates with the NREM sleep system, we need to discuss the common and different features of sleep and absences including an analysis of "loss of consciousness" in the two states.

Studies on the impairment of consciousness during absences (Blumenfeld, 2005; Stefan and Ramp, 2009) have revealed that it is far from global or uniform. It is different from patient to patient; and it may be fragmented by "pieces" of consciousness. The individually variable cortical pattern of activation/deactivation shown by the positive and negative blood oxygen level–dependent (BOLD) signals consistently supports this experience (Berman et al., 2010; Moeller et al., 2010; Szaflarski et al., 2010). The most commonly affected cortical functions are perception, cognition, and motor performance.

The variable and fragmentary distribution of functional deficits in different cortical functions, including consciousness, is in keeping with the spatially and temporally variable buildup of the normal sleep process, reflected by topographic differences in the development of slow waves, sleep spindles (Nir et al., 2011), and gamma bursts (Le Van Quyen et al., 2008).

This variability of the NREM sleep level parallels the asynchronous and uneven epileptic transformation of the bursting-mode activity in the corticothalamic system to SWDs.

The change in consciousness is far from identical during sleep and absences. First, there is an obvious motor inhibition during absences, whereas in sleep, at least during NREM, the motor output is intact. There is an ongoing mental activity when the sleeper is aroused, whereas no mental activity can be detected during absences. The differences in the electrocortical activity of sleep versus absences are even more complex. During NREM sleep there are more or less synchronized frontally dominant slow waves and central spindling, whereas during absences synchronous SWDs cover the whole scalp, and more so in the frontal region. The underlying event is a glutamatergic burst discharge in both the cortical and the thalamic relay cells during the "spike" component. The "wave" component used to be considered the sum of inhibitory postsynaptic potentials attributed to a GABAergic inhibitory process in the pyramidal cortical neurons. Steriade (2003c) later proposed a "disfacilitation" instead.

In contrast to NREM sleep, in which brain connectivity is reduced (Massimini et al., 2005), the functional connectivity during absences is higher, but less complex (Babloyantz and Destexhe, 1986).

Positron emission tomography (PET) studies have shown that both metabolic activity and blood flow are reduced during NREM sleep compared to resting wakefulness (Braun et al., 1997; Hofle et al., 1997; Maquet, 1997; Kajimura et al., 1999), probably because the hyperpolarized phase of the slow oscillation abolishes synaptic activity. The activation is low in all types of association cortices, whereas it is preserved in the primary sensory cortices. NREM sleep is a dynamic state compared to absences, involving several local changes and phasic events associated with the slow waves, spindling, vertex waves, and K complexes. All these microstructural components have specific dynamics explored by EEG–functional magnetic resonance imaging (fMRI) and source localization methods (Schabus et al., 2007; Czisch et al., 2009; Stern et al., 2011), revealing a dramatic reorganization of the brain connectivity architecture from wakefulness to NREM sleep.

Based upon PET studies, Raichle et al. (2001) first described a peculiar network (Fig. 2.6), which they called the resting state or default mode network (DMN).

Default Mode Network and Epilepsy

The existence of a major distributed functional network of the healthy brain typically associated with introspection, autobiographical memories, internal rumination, and self-referential processes engaged with past and future is established knowledge (Raichle et al., 2001). It is called the DMN. Major nodes of the DMN include the posterior cingulate/retrosplenial cortex, medial prefrontal cortex, and inferior parietal lobule (Buckner et al., 2008). There is a spatially coherent, low-frequency (<0.1 Hz) spontaneous fluctuation in the BOLD signal among the resting state nodes (Fig. 2.6).

EEG–fMRI studies have demonstrated a temporal association between interictal epileptiform discharges and activity changes in DMN nodes, revealing a deactivation (Archer a, Salek-Haddadi, Laufs, Fahoum a,b) or activation (Archer b) of the DMN network. In the studies in which resting state fMRI sessions with versus without the occurrence of spikes were

Default network (resting state)

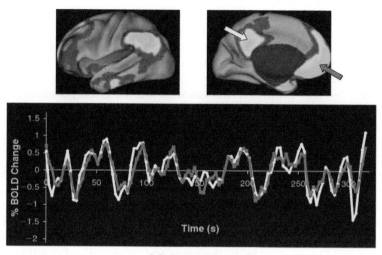

BOLD signal fluctuation

FIGURE 2.6   Top: The characteristic frontomedial and parietal regions of the dorsomedial nucleus. Bottom: The oscillation pattern connecting the distributed parallel functioning regions (in the resting state of the medial frontal and precuneal areas). BOLD, blood oxygen level–dependent. *After the work of Raichle, M.E., MacLeod, A.M., Snyder, A.Z., Powers, W.J., Gusnard, D.A., Shulman, G.L., 2001. A default mode of brain function. Proc. Natl. Acad. Sci. U.S.A 98(2), 676–682.*

compared, more network abnormalities were found in sessions containing interictal discharges (Centeno and Carmichael, 2014).

The direction of the relationship is not clear. Interictal epileptic discharge (IED) might cause DMN changes as suggested by the majority of publications. Certain brain states are more permissive for IEDs than others (this type of relationship is detailed in Chapter 1: IEDs and NREM sleep, and reactive slow waves within sleep). Lopes et al. (2014) measured functional connectivity before, during, and after IEDs of generalized and focal epilepsy patients. They found an increase in the connectivity before the occurrence of IEDs, suggesting that DMN connectivity change may facilitate IED generation. Therefore, the question whether IEDs are able to shape the DMN or conversely other intrinsic brain networks (e.g., the sleep–wake network) gate IEDs (as seen Chapter 1) has not been clarified.

The DMN appeared together with the emergence of aimless thinking and disappeared when the brain turned to goal-directed activities. It is linked to internal mental processes including day dreaming, free associations, and a free-floating awareness of the environment. In addition to the interindividually similar, stereotyped appearance of the DMN, it has been shown that, parallel to the BOLD switch related to DMN versus goal-directed networks, a spatially specific gamma-band activity can be detected as well (Raichle, 2010).

The work of Säman et al. has shown that when the DMN was tracked during the transition from wakefulness to slow-wave sleep and its further deepening, the contribution of the posterior cingulate cortex, the retrosplenial cortex, the parahippocampal gyrus, and the medial prefrontal cortex gradually decreased, paralleling the deepening of sleep.

Similar but less important changes were shown in the posterior cingulate and retrosplenial cortices during periods of increased sleep pressure in wakefulness (Ossandón et al., 2011).

During absences, transcranial Doppler ultrasonography of the middle cerebral artery has demonstrated a reduced blood flow (Nehlig et al., 1996), and single photon emission computerized tomography studies in experimental animals and humans revealed a decrease in blood flow in the cortex and its increase in the thalamus (Nehlig et al., 2004). Congruently, fluorodeoxyglucose–PET studies have shown a thalamic activation and a cortical deactivation (Bilo et al., 2010), and fMRI studies have revealed positive BOLD activation in the thalamus and patchy mixed positive–negative BOLD activation with negative preponderance over wide cortical fields (Fig. 2.7) (Aghakhani et al., 2004).

Archer et al. (2003) observed a deactivation in the posterior cingulate gyrus and in the bilateral parietal and anterior frontal regions during absences. Aghakhani et al. (2004) found an activation response in the thalamus in 80% of patients but an inconsistent pattern of activation and deactivation in the frontal and posterior areas. Later Gotman et al. (2005) performed a group analysis of absences, finding that the activations were most significant bilaterally in the thalamus and that there were activations in the mesial frontal region, in the bilateral insula, and in the cerebellum as well. The deactivations were surprisingly similar to the findings of Archer et al. (2003) and to the pattern of the DMN, especially in the posterior cingulate gyrus and the bilateral parietal and anterior frontal regions. Moeller et al. (2010) studied the activation pattern comparing the absences of one patient and absences of different patients as well. The BOLD spatial and temporal response patterns were very consistent across the discharges of one patient, whereas the results were variable in the absences of different patients. There was a consistent deactivation of the DMN some seconds before the start of an absence and an initial circumscribed frontal positive BOLD activation at its onset or shortly after. The DMN deactivation exceeded the duration of the absences (Fig. 2.8).

We can see that the functional neuroimaging studies have confirmed the existence of multiple local functional deficit zones in the cortex during absences; however, it is not clear if the fragmentary deficits of conscious awareness are or not related to them.

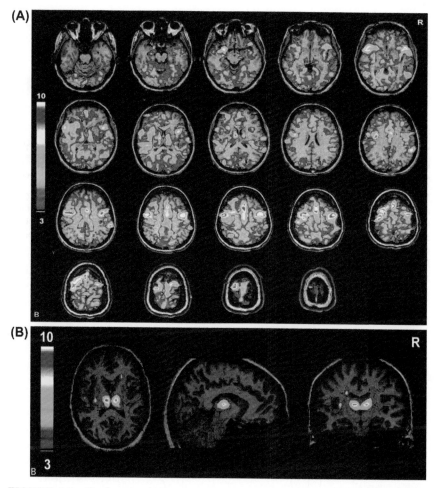

FIGURE 2.7 The functional MRI picture of absences (Aghakhani et al., 2004). Top row: Positive blood oxygen level–dependent (BOLD) activation of the thalami. Bottom: BOLD negative and BOLD positive patchy mosaic-like activation of the bilateral convexity.

Another feature of slow-wave sleep is the continuous alternation of cortical activation–deactivation (in time, not in space), approximately every 1000–1500 ms, consistent with the alternation of depolarized (up state) and hyperpolarized (down state) phases of <1 Hz slow-wave activity.

Concerning the consistent appearance of the DMN before absences, we propose that it may represent the precipitating drop in vigilance level evidenced by other methods. Carney and Jackson (2014) called it a "permissive cortical event" known to be required for the occurrence of a clinical absence and/or an EEG paroxysm.

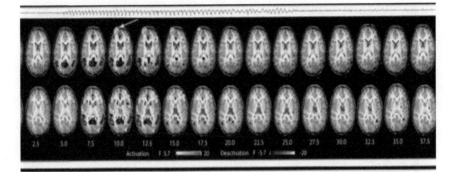

FIGURE 2.8   Sequences of blood oxygen level–dependent (BOLD) activation during an absence (captured every 2.5 s). Top: EEG pattern. The default mode network activation comes first (blue), then a right frontal focal activation (yellow) at 10 s is seen coincident with a positive BOLD activation (red) of the thalamus. At the same time, the patchy negative and positive spots appear over the frontal region. *NFLE*, nocturnal frontal lobe epilepsy. *From Moeller, F., LeVan, P., Muhle, H., Stephani, U., Dubeau, F., Siniatchkin, M., Gotman, J., 2010. Absence seizures: individual patterns revealed by EEG-fMRI. Epilepsia 51 (10), 2000–2010 with permission.*

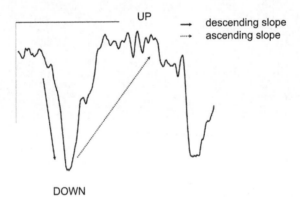

FIGURE 2.9   The slow oscillation consists of alternating depolarized (down) and hyperpolarized (up) states. During down states there are no fast rhythms; during up states there is abundant faster activity (from gamma to high frequencies).

The functional significance of the alternation between the sleep-related near-wake level activation during up states and the complete loss of activity during down states is unknown. Destexhe et al. (2007) have raised the question: "Are corticothalamic up states fragments of wakefulness?" and have argued supporting this possibility (Fig. 2.9). They have shown the similarity of the persistent depolarization during wakefulness versus the up states of <1-Hz slow oscillations in the cortical and thalamic relay neurons. Based upon their interpretation the short duration of the depolarization during up states does not allow gaining back conscious awareness, probably requiring a longer lasting uninterrupted activation. They have shown that the T-type Ca^{2+} channel-dependent bursts of action potentials that initiate each up state in the corticothalamic neurons might act as triggers for synaptic and cellular plastic processes in the corticothalamic networks. This is consistent with those behavioral experiments suggesting that slow-oscillation up states provide a context for the replay and possible consolidation of previous experiences.

The absence-related loss of contact with the environment may have multiple reasons. The bursting mode interrupts the flow of information toward the cortex and the inhibition or disfacilitation during the "wave" component involving the cortical association areas may compromise cortical elaboration. In addition, the invading SWDs may destroy the DMN, the substrate of the permanent, floating awareness of the environment, resulting in variable degrees of disturbances of contact during absences.

On the other hand, sensory stimuli may have an awakening/disruptive effect both in sleep and in absence seizures.

Gotman and Kostopoulos (2013) have raised the possibility that the "deactivation of the DMN may be fully or partially responsible for diminished self-awareness during spike-and-wave discharges, together with the presence of an abnormally active thalamus, and this may contribute to a partial blocking of sensory information reaching normally the cortex, thus reducing the awareness of the external world".

NON–RAPID EYE MOVEMENT SLEEP BURST-FIRING MODE AND ABSENCES SHARE A COMMON PHYSIOLOGICAL BACKGROUND (FIG. 2.10)

1. NREM sleep spindles originating in the burst-firing working mode may transform into SWDs under the influence of different changes in the system, including genetic or neurochemical effects. The key mechanism by which the physiological spindling of NREM sleep may switch to spike–wave paroxysms seems to be the mutual inhibition between RE neurons, regulating the level of the output inhibition exerted on the thalamic relay cells. When the output inhibition coming from the RE neurons is high (the intra-RE inhibition is low), the RE to thalamic relay cell inhibition would be more effective, leading to hypersynchronization in the form of spike–waves (Von Krosigk et al., 1993; Bal et al., 1995a,b; Huguenard and Prince, 1994; Sanchez-Vives et al., 1995; Kim et al., 1997).

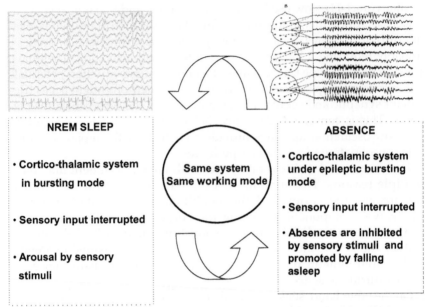

"Epilepsy and sleep are bedfellows" (M.Steriade)

FIGURE 2.10   Non–rapid eye movement (*NREM*) sleep burst-firing mode and absences share the same corticothalamic network. Top left: EEG of NREM sleep slow-wave activity. Top right: The ictal spike–wave activity of absences. Bottom: Comparison of the corticothalamic system working mode during NREM sleep (left) and absences (right).

2. Several sleep microstructural studies have evidenced that those phasic inputs pushing toward NREM (expressed by reactive slow waves) may promote absences/SWDs, whereas pure arousals, wakefulness, and REM sleep have a reverse, inhibiting effect on them (Halász, 1982; Terzano et al., 1989; Parrino et al., 2000; Halász et al., 2002a,b; Koutroumanidis et al., 2012).

References

Aghakhani, Y., Bagshaw, A.P., Bénar, C.G., Hawco, C., Andermann, F., Dubeau, F., Gotman, J., 2004. fMRI activation during spike and wave discharges in idiopathic generalized epilepsy. Brain 127 (Pt. 5), 1127–1144.

Archer, J.S., Abbott, D.F., Waites, A.B., Jackson, G.D., 2003. fMRI "deactivation" of the posterior cingulate during generalized spike and wave. Neuroimage 20 (4), 1915–1922.

Avoli, M., 2012. A brief history on the oscillating roles of thalamus and cortex in Absence seizures. Epilepsia 53 (5), 779–789.

Babloyantz, A., Destexhe, A., 1986. Low-dimensional chaos in an instance of epilepsy. Proc. Natl. Acad. Sci. U.S.A. 83 (10), 3513–3517.

Bal, T., von Krosigk, M., McCormick, D.A., 1995a. Role of the ferret perigeniculate nucleus in the generation of synchronized oscillations in vitro. J. Physiol. 483 (3), 665–685.

Bal, T., von Krosigk, M., McCormick, D.A., 1995b. Synaptic and membrane mechanisms underlying synchronized oscillations in the ferret LGN in vitro. J. Physiol. 483 (3), 641–663.

Bancaud, J., Talairach, J., Morel, P., Bresson, M., Bonis, A., Geie, S., et al., 1974. "Generalized" epileptic seizures elicited by electrical stimulation of the frontal lobe in man. Electroenceph. Clin Neurophsyiol 37, 275–282.

Beenhakker, M.P., Huguenard, J.R., 2009. Neurons that fire together also conspire together: is normal sleep circuitry hijacked to generate epilepsy? Neuron. 62 (5), 612–632.

Berman, R., Negishi, M., Vestal, M., Spann, M., Chung, M.H., Bai, X., Purcaro, M., Motelow, J.E., Danielson, N., Dix-Cooper, L., Enev, M., Novotny, E.J., Constable, R.T., Blumenfeld, H., 2010. Simultaneous EEG, fMRI, and behavior in typical childhood absence seizures. Epilepsia 51 (10), 2011–2022.

Bilo, L., Meo, R., de Leva, M.F., Vicidomini, C., Salvatore, M., Pappatà, S., 2010. Thalamic activation and cortical deactivation during typical absence status monitored using [^{18}F] FDG-PET: a case report. Seizure 19 (3), 198–201.

Blumenfeld, H., 2005. Consciousness and epilepsy: why are patients with absence seizures absent? Prog. Brain Res. 150, 271–286.

Blumenfeld, H., Klein, J.P., Schridde, U., Vestal, M., Rice, T., Khera, D.S., Bashyal, C., Giblin, K., Paul-Laughinghouse, C., Wang, F., Phadke, A., Mission, J., Agarwal, R.K., Englot, D.J., Motelow, J., Nersesyan, H., Waxman, S.G., Levin, A.R., 2008. Early treatment suppresses the development of spike-wave epilepsy in a rat model. Epilepsia 49 (3), 400–409.

Braun, A.R., Balkin, T.J., Wesenten, N.J., Carson, R.E., Varga, M., Baldwin, P., Selbie, S., Belenky, G., Herscovitch, P., 1997. Regional cerebral blood flow throughout the sleep-wake cycle. An H15 2 O PET study. Brain 120 (Pt 7), 1173–1197.

Buckner, R.L., Andrews-Hanna, J.R., Schacter, D.L., 2008. The brain's default network: anatomy, function, and relevance to disease. Ann. N. Y. Acad. Sci. 1124, 1–38.

Carney, P.W., Jackson, G.D., 2014. Insights into the mechanisms of absence seizure generation provided by EEG with functional MRI. Front. Neurol. 5, 162.

Centeno, M., Carmichael, D.W., 2014. Network connectivity in epilepsy: resting state fMRI and EEG-fMRI contributions. Front. Neurol. 5, 93.

Coenen, A.M., Drinkenburg, W.H., Peeters, B.W., Vossen, J.M., Van Luijtelaar, E.L., 1991. Absence epilepsy and the level of vigilance in rats of theWAG/Rij strain. Neurosci. Biobehav. Rev. 15 (2), 259–263.

Czisch, M., Wehrle, R., Stiegler, A., Peters, H., Andrade, K., Holsboer, F., Sämann, P.G., 2009. Acoustic oddball during NREM sleep: a combined EEG/fMRI study. PLoS One 4 (8), e6749.

Deleuze, C., Huguenard, J.R., 2006. Distinct electrical and chemical connectivity maps in the thalamic reticular nucleus: potential roles in synchronization and sensation. J. Neurosci. 26 (33), 8633–8645.

Destexhe, A., Hughes, S.W., Rudolph, M., Crunelli, V., 2007. Are corticothalamic 'up' states fragments of wakefulness? Trends Neurosci. 30 (7), 334–342.

Drinkenburg, W.H., Coenen, M.L., Vossen, J.M., van Luijtelaar, E.L., 1991. Spike-wave discharges and sleep-wake states in rats with absence epilepsy. Epilepsy Res. 9 (3), 218–224.

Ferri, R., Huber, R., Aricò, D., Drago, V., Rundo, F., Ghilardi, M.F., Massimini, M., Tononi, G., 2008. The slow-wave components of the cyclic alternating pattern (CAP) have a role in sleep-related learning processes. Neurosci. Lett. 432 (3), 228–231.

Gareri, P., Condorelli, D., Belluardo, N., Citraro, R., Barresi, V., Trovato-Salinaro, A., Mudò, G., Ibbadu, G.F., Russo, E., De Sarro, G., 2005. Antiabsence effects of carbenoxolone in two genetic animal models of absence epilepsy (WAG/Rij rats and lh/lh mice). Neuropharmacol 49 (4), 551–563.

Gigli, G.L., Calia, E., Marciani, M.G., Mazza, S., Mennuni, G., Diomedi, M., Terzano, M.G., Janz, D., 1992. Sleep microstructure and EEG epileptiform activity in patients with juvenile myoclonic epilepsy. Epilepsia 33 (5), 799–804.

Gloor, P., 1968. Generalized cortico-reticular epilepsies, some considerations on the pathophysiology of generalized bilaterally synchronous spike and wave discharge. Epilepsia 9 (3), 249–263.

Gloor, P., Fariello, R.G., 1988. Generalized epilepsy: some of its cellular mechanisms differ from those of focal epilepsy. Trends Neurosci. 11 (2), 63–68.

Gloor, P., Testa, G., Guberman, A., 1973. Brain-stem and cortical mechanisms in an animal model of generalized corticoreticular epilepsy. Trans. Am. Neurol. Assoc. 98, 203–205.

Gloor, P., Avoli, M., Kostopoulos, G., 1990. Thalamocortical relationships in generalized epilepsy with bilaterally synchronous spike-and-wave discharge. In: Avoli, M., Gloor, P., Kostopoulos, G., Naquet, R. (Eds.), Generalized Epilepsy: Neurobiological Approaches. MA Birkhauser, Boston.

Gotman, J., Kostopoulos, G., 2013. Absence seizures. In: Cavanna, A.E., Nani, A., Blumenfeld, H., Laureys, S. (Eds.), Neuroimaging of Consciousness. Springer-Verlag Berlin, Heidelberg, pp. 63–79.

Gotman, J., Grova, C., Bagshaw, A., Kobayashi, E., Aghakhani, Y., Dubeau, F., 2005. Generalized epileptic discharges show thalamocortical activation and suspension of the default state of the brain. Proc. Natl. Acad. Sci. U.S.A. 102 (42), 15236–15240.

Halász, P., 1982. The Role of Phasic Activation in Sleep Regulation and in Generalized Epilepsy with Spike-wave Pattern Academic Theses, Budapest.

Halász, P., Dévényi, É., 1974. Petit mal absence in night-sleep with special reference to transitional sleep and REM periods. Acta Med. Acad. Sci. Hung. 31 (1–2), 31–45.

Halász, P., Filakovszky, J., Vargha, A., Bagdy, G., 2002a. Effect of sleep deprivation on spike-wave discharges in idi-opathic generalised epilepsy: a 4x24 h continuous long term EEG monitoring study. Epilepsy Res. 51 (1–2), 123–132.

Halász, P., Terzano, M.G., Parrino, L., 2002b. Spike-wave discharge and the microstructure of sleep-wake continuum in idiopathic generalised epilepsy. Neurophysiol. Clin. 32 (1), 38–53.

Hofle, N., Paus, T., Reutens, D., Fiset, P., Gotman, J., Evans, A.C., Jones, B.E., 1997. Regional cerebral blood flow changes as a function of delta and spindle activity during slow wave sleep in humans. J. Neurosci. 17 (12), 4800–4808.

Holmes, M.D., Brown, M., Tucker, D.M., 2004. Are generalized seizures truly generalized? Evidence of localized mesial frontal and frontopolar discharges in absence. Epilepsia 45, 1568–1579.

Huguenard, J.R., McCormick, D.A., 2007. Thalamic synchrony and dynamic regulation of global forebrain oscillations. Trends Neurosci. 30 (7), 350–356.

Huguenard, J.R., Prince, D.A., 1994. Intrathalamic rhythmicity studied in vitro, nominal T current modulation causes robust antioscillatory effects. J. Neurosci. 14, 5485–5502.

Janz, D., 1974. Epilepsy and the sleeping-waking cycle. In: Vincken, P.J., Bruyn, G.W. (Eds.), Handbook of Clinical Neurology. The Epilepsies, vol. 15. North Holland, Amsterdam, The Netherlands, pp. 457–490.

Jasper, H.H., 1977. Wilder Penfield: his legacy to neurology. The centrencephalic system. Can. Med. Assoc. J 116 (12), 1371–1372.

Jasper, H.H., Droogleever-Fortuyn, J., 1974. Experimental studies of the functional anatomy of petit mal epilepsy. Res. Publ. Assoc. Nerv. Ment. Dis. 26, 272–298.

Kajimura, N., Uchiyama, M., Takayama, Y., Uchida, S., Uema, T., Kato, M., Sekimoto, M., Watanabe, T., Nakajima, T., Horikoshi, S., Ogawa, K., Nishikawa, M., Hiroki, M., Kudo, Y., Matsuda, M., Takahashi, K., 1999. Activity of midbrain reticular formation and neocortex during the progression of human non-rapid eye movement sleep. J. Neurosci. 19 (22), 10065–10073.

Kim, U.M., Sanchez-Vives, V., McCormick, D.A., 1997. Functional dynamics of GABAergic inhibition in the thalamus. Science 278 (5335), 130–134.

Klein, J.P., Khera, D.S., Nersesyan, H., Kimchi, E.Y., Waxman, S.G., Blumenfeld, H., 2004. Dysregulation of sodium channel expression in cortical neurons in a rodent model of absence epilepsy. Brain Res. 1000 (1–2), 102–109.

Kostopoulos, G.K., 2000. Spike-and-wave discharges of absence seizures as a transformation of sleep spindles: the continuing development of a hypothesis. Clin. Neurophysiol. 111 (Suppl. 2), S27–S38.

Kostopoulos, G., Gloor, P., Pellegrini, A., Gotman, J., 1981. A study of the transition from spindles to spike and wave discharge in feline generalized penicillin epilepsy: micro-physiological features. Exp. Neurol. 73 (1), 55–77.

Koutroumanidis, M., Tsiptsios, D., Kokkinos, V., Kostopoulos, G.K., 2012. Focal and generalized EEG paroxysms in childhood absence epilepsy: topographic associations and distinctive behaviors during the first cycle of non-REM sleep. Epilepsia 53 (5), 840–849.

Le Van Quyen, M., Bragin, A., Staba, R., Crépon, B., Wilson, C.L., Engel Jr., J., 2008. Cell type-specific firing during ripple oscillations in the hippocampal formation of humans. J. Neurosci. 28 (24), 6104–6110.

Lopes, R., Moeller, F., Besson, P., Ogez, F., Szurhaj, W., Leclerc, X., Siniatchkin, M., Chipaux, M., Derambure, P., Tyvaert, L., 2014. Study on the relationships between intrinsic functional connectivity of the default mode network and transient epileptic activity. Front. Neurol. 5, 201.

Manning, J.P., Richards, D.A., Leresche, N., Crunelli, V., Bowery, N.G., 2004. Cortical-area specific block of genetically determined absence seizures by ethosuximide. Neuroscience 123 (1), 5–9.

Maquet, P., 1997. Positron emission tomography studies of sleep and sleep disorders. J. Neurol. 244 (S1), S23–S28.

Massimini, M., Ferrarelli, F., Huber, R., Esser, S.K., Singh, H., Tononi, G., 2005. Breakdown of cortical effective connectivity during sleep. Science 309 (5744), 2228–2232.

McCromick, D.A., Bal, T., 1997. Sleep and arousal: thalamocortical mechanisms. Ann. Rev. Neurosci. 20, 185–215.

Meeren, H., Pijn, J.P., Luijtelaar, G., Coenen, A., Lopes da Silva, F.H., 2002. Cortical focus drives widespread corticothalamic networks during spontaneous absence seizures. J. Neurosci 22, 1480–1495.

Meeren, H., van Luijtelaar, G., Lopes da Silva, F., Coenen, A., 2005. Evolving concepts on the pathophysiology of absence seizures: the cortical focus theory. Arch. Neurol. 62 (3), 371–376.

Moeller, F., LeVan, P., Muhle, H., Stephani, U., Dubeau, F., Siniatchkin, M., Gotman, J., 2010. Absence seizures: individual patterns revealed by EEG-fMRI. Epilepsia 51 (10), 2000–2010.

Nehlig, A., Vergnes, M., Waydelich, R., Hirsch, E., Charbonne, R., Marescaux, C., Seylaz, J., 1996. Absence seizures induce a decrease in cerebral blood flow: human and animal data. J. Cereb. Blood Flow. Metab. 16 (1), 147–155.

Nehlig, A., Valenti, M.P., Thiriaux, A., Hirsch, E., Marescaux, C., Namer, I.J., 2004. Ictal and interictal perfusion variations measured by SISCOM analysis in typical childhood absence epilepsy. Epileptic Disord. 6 (4), 247–253.

Niedermeyer, E., 1967. Über auslösende Mechanismen von Kramfpotentialen bei centrenphaler Epilepsie. Nervenarzt 38, 72–74.

Niedermeyer, E., 1972. The Generalized Epilepsies: A Clinical Electroencephalographic Study. C.C. Thomas, Springfield, Ill, USA.

Niedermeyer, E., 1991. Awakening epilepsy ('Aufwach-Epilepsie') revisited. Epilepsy Res. 2, 37–42.

Niedermeyer, E., Laws, E.R., walker, E.A., 1969. Depth EEG findings in epileptic patients with generalized spike-wave complexes. Arch. Neurol. 21, 51–58.

Nir, Y., Staba, R.J., Andrillon, T., Vyazovskiy, V.V., Cirelli, C., Fried, I., Tononi, G., 2011. Regional slow waves and spindles in human sleep. Neuron 70 (1), 153–169.

Ossandón, T., Jerbi, K., Vidal, J.R., Bayle, D.J., Henaff, M.A., Jung, J., Minotti, L., Bertrand, O., Kahane, P., Lachaux, J.P., 2011. Transient suppression of broadband gamma power in the default-mode network is correlated with task complexity and subject performance. J. Neurosci. 31 (41), 14521–14530.

Parrino, L., Smerieri, A., Spaggiari, M.C., Terzano, M.G., 2000. Cyclic alternating pattern (CAP) and epilepsy: how a physiological rhythm modulates a pathological event. Clin. Neurophysiol. 111 (Suppl. 2), S39–S46.

Passouant, P., 1971. Absence or petit mal. Clinical and physiopathological problems. Rev. Esp. Ot. Neurocir. 29 (167), 11–28.

Pavlova, M.K., Shea, S.A., Scheer, F.A.J.L., Bromfield, E.B., 2009. Is there a circadian variation of epileptiform abnormalities in idiopathic generalized epilepsy? Epilepsy Behav. 16 (3), 461–467.

Raichle, M.E., 2010. Two views of brain function. Trends Cogn. Sci. 14 (4), 180–190.

Raichle, M.E., MacLeod, A.M., Snyder, A.Z., Powers, W.J., Gusnard, D.A., Shulman, G.L., 2001. A default mode of brain function. Proc. Natl. Acad. Sci. U.S.A. 98 (2), 676–682.

Rajna, P., Lona, C., 1989. Sensory stimulation for inhibition of epileptic seizures. Epilepsia 30 (2), 168–174.

Sanchez-Vives, M.V., Bal, T., McCormick, D.A., 1995. Properties of GABAergic inhibition in the ferret LGNd contributing to the generation of synchronized oscillations. Soc. Neurosci. Abst. 21, 11.

Schabus, M., Dang-Vu, T.T., Albouy, G., Balteau, E., Boly, M., Carrier, J., Darsaud, A., Degueldre, C., Desseilles, M., Gais, S., Phillips, C., Rauchs, G., Schnakers, C., Sterpenich, V., Vandewalle, G., Luxen, A., Maquet, P., 2007. Hemodynamic cerebral correlates of sleep spindles during human non-rapid eye movement sleep. Proc. Natl. Acad. Sci. U.S.A. 104 (32), 13164–13169.

Slaght, S.J., Leresche, N., Deniau, J., Crunelli, M.V., Charpier, S., 2002. Activity of thalamic reticular neurons during pontaneous genetically determined spike and wave discharges. J. Neurosci. 22 (6), 2323–2334.

Smyk, M.K., Coenen, A.M.L., Lewandowski, M.H., van Luijtelaar, G., 2011. Endogenous rhythm of absence epilepsy: relationship with general motor activity and sleep-wake states. Epilepsy Res. 93 (2–3), 120–127.

Stefan, H., Ramp, S., 2009. Current clinical-neurophysiological findings in absence epilepsies. Nervenarzt 80 (4), 378–385.

Steriade, M., 2003a. Neuronal Substrates of Sleep and Epilepsy. Cambridge University Press, pp. 95–171.

Steriade, M., 2003b. Neuronal Substrates of Sleep and Epilepsy. Cambridge University Press, pp. 336–337.

Steriade, M., 2003c. Neuronal Substrates of Sleep and Epilepsy. Cambridge University Press, p. 357.

Steriade, M., Deschênes, M., Domich, L., Mulle, C., 1985. Abolition of spindle oscillations in thalamic neurons disconnected from nucleus reticularis thalami. J. Neurophysiol. 54 (6).

Stern, J.M., Caporro, M., Haneef, Z., Yeh, H.J., Buttinelli, C., Lenartowicz, A., Mumford, J.A., Parvizi, J., Poldrack, R.A., 2011. Functional imaging of sleep vertex sharp transients. Clin. Neurophysiol. 122 (7), 1382–1386.

Stevens, J.R., Kodama, H., Lonsbury, B., Mills, L., 1971. Ultradian characteristics of spontaneous seizures discharges recorded by radio telemetry in man. Electroencephalogr. Clin. Neurophysiol. 31 (4), 313–325.

Suntsova, N., Kumar, S., Guzman-Marin, R., Alam, M.N., Szymusiak, R., McGinty, D., 2009. A role for the preoptic sleep promoting system in absence epilepsy. Neurobiol. Dis. 36 (1), 126–141.

Szaflarski, J.P., DiFrancesco, M., Hirschauer, T., Banks, C., Privitera, M.D., Gotman, J., Holland, S.K., 2010. Cortical and subcortical contributions to absence seizure onset examined with EEG/fMRI. Epilepsy Behav. 18 (4), 404–413.

Tenney, J.R., Glauser, T.A., 2013. The current state of absence epilepsy: can we have your attention? Epilepsy Curr. 13 (3), 135–140.

Terzano, M.G., Parrino, L., Anelli, S., Halász, P., 1989. Modulation of generalized spike-and-wave discharges during sleep by cyclic alternating pattern. Epilepsia 30 (6), 772–781.

Tomka, I., 1985. Circadian features of petit mal epilepsy. EEG-EMG Z. für Elektroenzephalogr. Elektromyogr. Verwandte Geb. 16 (1), 10–16.

Tükel, K., Jasper, H., 1952. The electroencephalogram in parasagittal lesions. Electroencephalogr. Clin. Neurophysiol. 4 (4), 481–494.

Von Krosigk, M., Bal, T., McCormick, D.A., 1993. Cellular mechanisms of a synchronized oscillation in the thalamus. Science 261 (5119), 361–364.

Westmijse, I., Ossenblok, P., Gunning, B., van Luijtelaar, G., 2009. Onset and propagation of spike and slow wave discharges in human absence epilepsy: a MEG study. Epilepsia 50 (12), 2538–2548.

Williams, D., 1965. The thalamus and epilepsy. Brain 88 (3), 539–556.

Zarowski, M., Loddenkemper, T., Vendrame, M., Alexopoulos, A.V., Wyllie, E., Kothare, S.V., 2011. Circadian distribution and sleep/wake patterns of generalized seizures in children. Epilepsia 52 (6), 1076–1083.

Autosomal Dominant Nocturnal Frontal Lobe and Nocturnal Frontal Lobe Epilepsy as System Epilepsies of the Ascending Cholinergic Arousal System

Nocturnal frontal lobe epilepsy (NFLE) is a specific epilepsy syndrome; its relationship with the rest of the frontal lobe epilepsies is not clear. It was first described as a sleep disorder called "paroxysmal nocturnal dystonia" (Lugaresi et al., 1986); and the epileptic nature of the seizures has been recognized after several years of clinical research. The seizures occur usually in non–rapid eye movement (NREM) sleep, clustering nightly and appearing just occasionally in the waking state, either in a form similar to that in sleep or as generalized tonic–clonic seizures. The attacks may appear in early childhood, persisting until adulthood, or in young adulthood. There is a male predisposition. The seizure semiology is variable, regarding both symptoms and severity.

NFLE patients have sporadic seizures of unknown origin. A minority of them have mutations of the nicotinic acetylcholine receptor subunits (Scheffer et al., 1995) and the related acetylcholinergic pathways. The electroclinical symptoms of the two groups [autosomal dominant nocturnal frontal lobe epilepsy (ADNFLE) and NFLE] are identical irrespective of their genetic origin (Provini et al., 1999). The labeling of the lesional cases representing a distinct group is important in the classification of NFLE (we will come back to this later).

Regardless of their complexity, different EEG/EMG/autonomic and behavioral signs of arousal (Bisulli et al., 2010) precede these seizures.

THE SYMPTOMS OF AROUSAL/ALARM/FRENETIC PANIC DURING SEIZURES: A PARALLELISM OF NFLE AND AROUSAL PARASOMNIAS

NFLE seizures are usually described as "hypermotor" because their most conspicuous feature is a movement storm, but they may manifest in several forms. In an increasing order of complexity, seemingly spontaneous fragments of simple sleep-related movements related to arousals without awakening; motor, autonomic, and emotional phenomena; frenetic alarm; and panic occur.

Derry et al. (2009) have reinvestigated the symptoms of video EEG–detected seizures in 63 NFLE patients and compared them with 57 arousal parasomnia (AP) events. They identified three fundamental patterns; 79% of the registered events contained more than one of them. The basic patterns were:

1. "Simple arousal behavior": This was the first or only element of 92% of the events, including eye opening, head lifting, staring and face rubbing, yawning, stretching, moaning, or mumbling.
2. "Nonagitated motor behavior" (72%): This included sitting forward, manipulating nearby objects, and an exploring (orienting) behavior.

Standing and walking only occasionally occurred in the electrode-mounted patients. The facial expression was impassive or perplexed and coherent speech fragments occurred.

3. "Distressed emotional behavior" (51%): Signs of fear and anguish were indicated by the facial expression and speech content. The patients sat or stood up, screaming and expressing frantic behavior. Attempts to restrain evoked an aggressive response.

The comparison of NFLE and AP-related events in the Derry study showed that 79% of AP events and 49% of NFLE seizures began with an arousal. Sixty-five percent of the AP events were followed by manifestations that were more dramatic. Tachycardia was a prominent feature in both groups.

Thirty-nine percent of the events were triggered by external (noise) or internal (cough or snore) stimuli in the AP group, whereas a trigger could be identified in just 8% of NFLE seizures.

In the NFLE group environmental interactions were present in only 11% of seizures and coherent speech was rare; it was a frenetic and not an interactive type, if present.

APs were terminated by NREM sleep in 74%, whereas 88% of NFLE seizures had an awakening effect.

One may draw several lessons from this study. The symptoms of NFLE seizures and AP events are astonishingly similar and they follow a parallel severity order. A typical common feature is a behavioral and autonomic arousal culminating in the third (distressed emotional behavior) pattern, what we call "hypermotor" in NFLE seizures and "night terrors" in AP. The external or internal triggering factors and communication with the environment were more frequent in AP compared to NFLE.

After this study the previous classification of AP events by Broughton (1968) into "confusional arousals," "sleepwalking" or "somnambulism," and "sleep terrors" seems to be outworn; rather, speaking about a continuum of both AP and seizure symptoms manifesting in different complexities holds more true. The striking similarity of NFLE and AP symptoms suggests a shared arousal-related mechanism (consistent with Broughton's denominating term "arousal parasomnia"), regardless of the epileptic or nonepileptic origin. The genetic links of NFLE and AP established in the meanwhile (Bisulli et al., 2010) support a shared brain mechanism of these two disorders as well.

Another aspect of the Derry study is that in the light of the data provided, the usual simple description of NFLE seizures as hypermotor does not catch the essence. The increasing complexity of the seizures, from fragments of plain arousal movements through nonagitated motor phenomena to severe alarm behavior with emotional expressions, may reflect different degrees of arousal with consistent behavioral manifestations.

The concept of a shared arousal mechanism would integrate the seemingly different types of motor, emotional, and autonomic manifestations of the two conditions.

NFLE AND THE DYNAMICS OF SLEEP MICROSTRUCTURE

Arousability and reactivity to sensory stimuli are essential features of sleep, differentiating it from coma, keeping the sleeper in contact with the environment. Thus, arousal from sleep has an important biological function, serving reversibility and as an alarm function awakening the sleeper in case of danger.

Sleep is scattered with variable-degree microarousals. These arousals used to be considered harmful, disturbing the sleep. The better understanding of sleep microstructure has highlighted the sleep-regulating role of arousals (Halász et al., 2004; Halász and Bódizs, 2013).

In the framework of the cyclic alternating pattern (CAP) system, phasic events without behavioral manifestations have been considered inherent parts of the dynamic sleep organization, making a microcyclicity of sleep. The CAP cycle consists of activation (A) and background (B) periods. The subtypes of the CAP A phase (A1, A2, A3) represent responses to external or internal stimuli congruent with the level of homeostatic pressure. A3 and partially A2 reflect microshifts toward rapid eye movement (REM) sleep or waking, whereas A1 is consistent with a tendency toward NREM sleep. The proper term for subtypes would be "activation with arousal (A3) or antiarousal (A1) features."

Sleep-related seizures linked to microarousals are the identifying manifestations of NFLE (Zucconi et al., 2000). However, the exact relationship with the CAP A phase is not quite clear. In the study of Parrino et al. (2012) more than 60% of NFLE attacks occurred in slow-wave sleep and 28% in stage 2. In the studies of Derry and Montagna most of them occurred during stage 2 NREM sleep (Derry et al., 2006; Montagna et al., 2008).

The frequency of seizures during the night was the highest in the first sleep cycles and it followed the homeostatic decay of slow-wave sleep across the night. The time, the rate, the number, and the duration of the CAP cycles, especially the rate of CAP A, were all elevated in NFLE patients compared to normal controls (Halász et al., 2013), pointing to a continuously higher level of activation during NREM sleep, suggested also by the obvious arousal-related motor elements of seizures. It is not clear whether these activation phenomena are causes or consequences of the seizures; however, the increased CAP rate, the increased frequency of CAP responses, and the sleep instability of NFLE patients favor the first possibility.

THE EPILEPTOGENIC MUTATION OF THE ACETYLCHOLINE RECEPTOR UNDERLIES THE HYPERSENSITIVITY OF THE AROUSAL SYSTEM IN ADNFLE

A familial clustering of NFLE cases has long been observed, and in 1995, Scheffer et al. described the familial variant of the disorder, called ADNFLE. The underlying cause was the mutation of the nicotinic acetylcholine (ACh) receptor (nAChR) a4 (*CHRNA4*) and b2 (*CHRNB2*) subunits on the 20q13 and 15q24 chromosomes. Additional gene mutations, affecting the nAChR and the related ACh pathways (Rozycka et al., 2003; Hildebrand et al., 2015; Weltzin et al., 2016), including the potassium sodium-activated channel subfamily T member 1 (*KCNT1*) and DEP domain-containing protein 5 (*DEPDC5*) (Kurahashi and Hirosi, 2002), have been described since. Interestingly, in Chinese ADNFLE patients the ACh-receptor gene mutations, which are causative in Caucasians, seem not to be involved (Chen et al., 2015).

ADNFLE patients with a clarified genotype represent a small minority of NFLE cases, carrying the same phenotypical features (Provini et al., 1999). The hint to finding a genetic etiology also in the sporadic NFLE population came from Liu et al. (2011), who verified the mutation of nAChR gene *CHRNB2* in Chinese nonfamilial NFLE patients.

ACh has an important role in the activation of the frontal cortex during arousals (Muzur et al., 2002), where the thalamus and the cortex are key structures. They are rich in cholinergic fibers originating from the nucleus basalis of Meynert, providing a most robust cholinergic input. Not only transsynaptic, but also nonsynaptic, ACh release is to be taken into account (Descarries et al., 1997). The presence of mutant nAChRs in ADNFLE suggests a pathological cholinergic arousal system in these patients. The mutant receptors of ADNFLE favor the frontal cortex, the thalamus, and the mesencephalic tegmentum, the last two structures belonging to the ascending arousal system (Han et al., 2000). A statistically significant increase in nAChR density was observed in ADNFLE patients in a region involving the mesencephalon, an adjacent part of the diencephalon (superior area of the epithalamus), and the cerebellum (Picard et al., 2006). The finding of an increased number of nAChRs in the regions of the epithalamus (medial habenular area) and the interpeduncular nucleus (IPN) is particularly interesting in the context of sleep disorders. These structures are parts of the limbic system outflow into the brain stem (Haun et al., 1992). They are linked by the fasciculus retroflexus, a cholinergic projection from the medial habenula to the IPN. The IPN projects to the ventral tegmental area and to the reticular and tegmental brainstem nuclei, particularly to the laterodorsal tegmental nucleus (LDT), which is part of the ascending cholinergic reticular activating system involved in the regulation of arousal. The IPN has important projections to the mediodorsal thalamic nucleus, which projects to the prefrontal cortex. The IPN is involved in the sleep–wake cycle primarily through its connections with the LDT, releasing ACh into the thalamus during NREM sleep at the time of arousals. This ACh release triggers an activated awake state in the corticothalamic system. Thus, any change or lesion affecting the IPN could result in arousal disorders. The increased sensitivity of the mutant receptors (gain of function) causes increased activation of the frontal cortex through the corticothalamic connections (Picard et al., 2006). In nAChR B2 subunit gene–knockout mice the frequency of microarousals in NREM decreased (Léna et al., 2004).

Based upon the aforementioned data we may assume that in ADNFLE, the hyperfunctioning mesopontine cholinergic pathway chronically over-activates the LDT and the mediodorsal thalamic nucleus. The consequent arousals result in epileptic and nonepileptic arousal-linked events.

NFLE seizures were believed to be *preceded* by arousals; however, we rather propose them to be activation/arousal responses themselves. The pathological motor, emotional, and autonomic behaviors involve a partial arousal, during which the frontal dorsolateral cognitive functioning is deactivated by the persistent partial sleep, reflected by a frontal convexity slow-wave EEG.

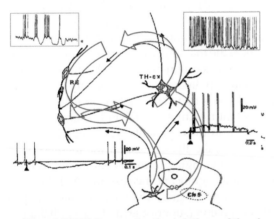

Absence Epilepsy (red) is the epileptic variation of the burst-firing working mode of the the cortico-thalamic system otherwise producing sleep spindles and slow waves

The ADNFLE (blue) is the manifestation of the epileptically facilitated frontal arousal

AE and ADFNLE are epileptic variations of the sleep induction and arousal

FIGURE 3.1 This schema shows the antagonistic functional networks of sleep and arousal systems as substrates of absence epilepsy and nocturnal frontal lobe epilepsy. *Red network*: The burst-firing working mode of the corticothalamic system during non–rapid eye movement (NREM) sleep. *Blue network*: The reciprocal antagonistic ascending arousal system. These systems are of utmost importance in regulating the sleep–wake balance. The balance is shifted toward NREM sleep in absence epilepsy (AE), where the burst-firing function is epileptically facilitated and the sleep-promoting antiarousal phasic microshift (cyclic alternating pattern A1) gates the ictal events. The balance is shifted toward arousal in autosomal dominant nocturnal frontal lobe epilepsy (*ADNFLE*), because of the gain-type mutation of the acetylcholine receptor function making the arousal system oversensitive to arousing inputs. *Ch S*, cholinergic neuron in the mesencephalic ascending arousal system providing the RE neurons with inhibitory innervation to the thalamocortical relay cells producing excitatory impulses; *RE*, thalamic reticular nucleus neuron; *TH-cx*, thalamocortical neuron. (After Itier and Bertrand, 2002)

BRAIN MECHANISMS UNDERLYING THE EPILEPTIC AND NONEPILEPTIC PATHOLOGICAL AROUSAL REACTIONS DURING SLEEP IN NFLE AND AROUSAL PARASOMNIA

The clinical similarities of NFLE and AP, their common relation with the sleep process, as well as their genetic link have suggested a common pathomechanism (Bisulli et al., 2010; Halász et al., 2012). Our understanding of the nature of sleep has very much changed by now. Its global nature has been challenged by those data pointing to the existence of local/regional features of sleep and wake states. In some neurologic conditions, the elements of different vigilance states occur simultaneously, e.g., REM sleep behavior disorder (often connected to Parkinson disease) manifests in motor activity during REM sleep. The recognition of the parallel presence of mixed features led to the notion of dissociated states (Mahowald, 2002). APs fit quite well into the state dissociation concept, being composite conditions with a "Janus face," presenting waking and sleeping behaviors and phenomena together. Experimental works proving the existence of sleeping cortical columns among waking ones have importantly contributed to the local sleep concept (Krueger et al., 1995). Another approach has revealed local differences in the delta power (local delta sleep increase) after the utilization of specific functions preceding the night of the investigation (Kattler et al., 1994). The alternating sleep of the two hemispheres discovered in dolphins and other aquatic mammals (Mukhametov et al., 1977; Lyamin et al., 2008) has confirmed the possibility of simultaneously existing mixed waking and sleeping regions in the brain occurring in certain sleep conditions and circumstances.

Two important publications have provided congruent objective evidence for such dissociated states in AP patients. Bassetti et al. (2000) reported a single photon emission computerized tomography study in a man with AP, nicely demonstrating a clear state dissociation: the activation of the thalamocingulate pathways in line with persisting deactivation of the frontodorsal region during a nocturnal AP episode.

Almost the same was demonstrated by Terzaghi et al. (2009) in a patient under invasive presurgical evaluation for epilepsy having a history of AP episodes. They were lucky to observe an AP event with implanted electrodes. During this event occurring in NREM sleep, the frontal convexity presented the usual slow-wave activity of NREM sleep while the cingular gyrus emanated wake-like activity.

A similar dissociation mechanism may underlie the sleep events of NFLE and AP.

The Role of Dissociated States During Sleep and Wakefulness in the Pathophysiology of Ictal and Postictal Automatisms

A special semiology feature of epileptic seizures is the development of automatisms, commonly observed in mesiotemporal and frontal lobe epilepsies. Because they represent the lobar functions, the symptoms of frontal and temporal automatisms are different. Their pathomechanism is far from clear; both epileptic excitation and postictal exhaustion may induce them. In the latter case, the exhaustion of certain cortical regions may disengage the activity of others. These kinds of automatisms represent inhibited functions, which would disengage because of the inactivation of the suppressing structure. In both variants—epileptic excitation or liberation—a ready set (stereotypically identical in each seizure) of a sensory, motor, or emotional pattern or "package" emerges. It may often be recognized as a mosaic of normal behavior, which appears without function (unduly and inadequately in the given situation) and with no awareness in the affected individual.

Does sleep have something to do with all these? It has long been noticed that sleep favors automatisms. Textbooks used to consider a disturbance of consciousness a prerequisite of automatisms; however, this supposition has been challenged by those automatisms observed in nondominant side seizures in fully alert patients (Ebner et al., 1995). This observation makes the idea that a decrease in vigilance level causes sleep-related automatisms rather ambiguous.

Discussing the local features of sleep, we could see in this book that local sleep may develop during wakefulness and, conversely, local wakefulness may appear during sleep, especially in pathological conditions (sleep disorders). Local sleep means that some cortical regions are awake in line with other regions sleeping at the same time. This pattern is called the dissociated state, explaining several pathological phenomena related to sleep (Mahowald and Schenk, 1992). Does this mechanism enlighten the development of automatisms as well?

This chapter highlights the similar pathomechanisms of NFLE and APs. The prefrontal cortex is one of the specific regions decreasing its activity during slow-wave sleep (SWS) compared to wakefulness, contributing to the lack of cognition in NREM sleep. One of the main reasons for the development of dissociative states during and after awakening might be the persistence of sleep in the prefrontal region, resulting in the temporary coexistence of sleep and wakefulness in the same brain. In such situations, there are automatic responses to the environment. There is no full alertness, no remembrance, nor recall of the occurrences and sophisticated contents, even less so than of dreams when awakening from REM sleep. This dissociation of the prefrontal cortex from the rest of the cortical regions may explain the lack of conscious control over the autonomic symptoms related to awakening, which then may be perceived as signs of a severe danger leading to panic and escape. Similar dissociation may occur in the arousal system and its frontal cortical projection in ADNFLE, characterized by a pathological shift toward arousal due to the epileptogenic mutations of the ACh-receptor structures.

Is this dissociation/liberation mechanism valid also in awake seizures or in the case of postictal automatisms? According to its definition, a postictal automatism is caused by the seizure-related exhaustion of a cortical region carrying an inhibitory function. This may lead to temporary disengagement (liberation) symptoms. Also, ictal automatisms may be underlain by the interference of seizure activity with some functions—including inhibiting ones—of the associated regions (e.g., in decremental seizures there is an important and widespread depolarization wave), resulting in liberation phenomena. Englot et al. (2010) have suggested that the disturbance of consciousness and the related bilateral slow-wave activity in wide regions of the association cortex seen in temporal lobe seizures would be caused by the epileptic excitation of the temporal lobes inhibiting the arousal system. An arousal-inhibiting function of the thalamus has been explored (Giber et al., 2015). It is possible that the poorly understood diaschisis phenomenon newly rediscovered by metabolic imaging methods (Carrera and Tononi, 2014) has similar causes.

These data suggest that state dissociation is a general phenomenon beyond the field of sleep and wakefulness. This broader sense of state dissociation could provide a better understanding and integration for the epileptic and nonepileptic automatisms than the liberation hypotheses (Llinas, 2002; Tassinari et al., 2005), which do not seem always appropriate.

Although the riddle of epileptic automatisms has always challenged epilepsy researchers, no up-to-date interpretation of this common symptom has been found. Under the source light of research, epileptic automatisms and the supposed underlying dissociative mechanisms should move from the group of curiosities as important factors of epileptic seizure semiology. The exploration of epileptic automatisms could become the driving force of the understanding of hierarchic brain organization, which has been an outstanding focus of many excellent brain researchers.

IS NFLE, OR "SLEEP-RELATED HYPERMOTOR EPILEPSY"[1], A HOMOGENEOUS SYNDROME WITH HETEROGENEOUS ETIOLOGICAL FACTORS?

The seizure semiology analysis of symptomatic NFLE cases allows some functional–anatomical grouping of the seizures. Those seizures that are linked to the arousal/alarm/fear/frightened behavior line followed by an

---

[1] A consensus conference discussing the different etiology and symptomatological and sleep-related aspects of NFLE proposed changing the name of the syndrome to "sleep-related hypermotor epilepsy" (SHE). The conclusions of the task force conference were published in 2016 (Tinuper et al., 2016).

NFLE - seizures from the mediobasal surface

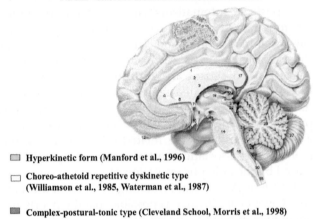

☐ **Hyperkinetic form (Manford et al., 1996)**

☐ **Choreo-athetoid repetitive dyskinetic type**
(Williamson et al., 1985, Waterman et al., 1987)

▨ **Complex-postural-tonic type (Cleveland School, Morris et al., 1998)**

FIGURE 3.2   The assumed relationship between different frontal territories of the medial and orbitofrontal surface and seizure symptoms in nocturnal frontal lobe epilepsy (*NFLE*).

escape activity might make up one subgroup. The symptoms of another potential subgroup with motor symptoms as repetitive automatisms (pelvic thrusting, pedaling, choreoathetoid and ballistic movements) and dystonic posturing might derive from the frontostriatal circuits. Seizures originating near the medial supplementary area presenting more tonic posturing constitute a third group, whereas intensive, fast, repetitive hypermotor elements have been observed in a fourth group of seizures related to the orbitofrontal and anterior–medial region (Fig. 3.2) (Manford et al., 1996). The involvement of the arousal system and of the ancient motor systems is the most consistent system-epileptic feature of sleep-related epilepsies (SREs). The seizures involving the arousal/alarm/panic line may have immediate and long-lasting consequences on the entire stress system. This important aspect has remained unexplored.

The diversity of the seizure manifestations could purely reflect the affected anatomical site (of the seizure onset or the propagation to the symptomatogenic zone) regardless of the etiology, e.g., a genetic hypersensitivity of the cholinergic arousal system or a frontal lobe lesion. Another hub of controversies affects the heterogeneity of the MRI and EEG findings. Earlier, at the "paroxysmal nocturnal dystonia" phase, and also later, when the large reviews about NFLE were published (Oldani et al., 1996; Provini et al., 1999), the interictal epileptic discharges were deemed to be minimal or absent even during seizures, and also (but less so) during sleep. Later, when the dysgenetic lesions came more to light and it turned out that there was a distinct specific MRI picture of a certain cortical dysplasia type, the epileptic EEG correlates were also better understood (Palmini et al., 1995). However, we still do not know whether we are indeed dealing with different or the same patient population.

The analysis of the frontal lesional epilepsy group has resulted in interesting data regarding sleep dependency as well as the frequency and severity of IEDs. Nobili et al. (2009) analyzed 303 drug-resistant epilepsy patients who had become seizure free after resective surgery. They correlated the feature of sleep relatedness with the resection sites and histology results. Thirty-nine patients (12.8%) had SRE. The higher occurrence of sleep-related attacks correlated with frontal onset and type II focal cortical dysplasia (FCD), whereas low seizure frequency correlated with other types of FCD, glioneural tumors, and hippocampal sclerosis. The only variable having a statistically significant link with SRE, increasing by 14-fold the chance of it, was type II FCD. It could also be concluded that irrespective of its site (even extrafrontal), the Taylor type II dysplasia, especially IIb, increased the risk of epileptic seizures during NREM sleep (Nobili et al., 2009; Tassi et al., 2012). In the FCD type II patients, localized rhythmic or pseudorhythmic spikes or polyspikes (brushes) and localized brief low-voltage fast activity were prevalent during NREM sleep. The brushes were highly (76%) associated with Taylor FCD type IIb lesions. The resection of these lesions produced an Engel class I outcome in 83% of patients remaining seizure free for long (Tassi et al., 2012).

Characterizing the corticographic features of dysplastic cortices, Palmini et al. (1995) described high-level "intrinsic epileptogenicity." The nearly continuous or recurrent periodic discharges switched to and fro between the interictal and the ictal state. This type of extreme epileptic activity has hardly occurred in other dysgenetic epilepsy conditions. The epileptic activity was restricted to the site of the MRI lesion, not influencing wider cortical regions. The complete surgical removal of the lesion defined by imaging, together with the resection of the overlapping discharging area, has ensured excellent surgical outcome.

A most interesting feature of the dysgenetic FCD type II lesions is the intrinsic epileptogenicity of the dysplastic lesion. Its electrographic reflection is of a variable degree, but continuous near-ictal-level epileptic excitation is intensified by NREM sleep (Palmini et al., 1995; Cordeiro et al., 2015), affecting both the interictal and the ictal activity. There is typically no spread and progression to generalized seizures (at least in adults), rather, the seizures remain in a circumscribed region. They constitute a very dynamic local interictal/ictal cycling of focalized seizure clusters, with the maintenance of a focal ictal susceptibility.

The special intrinsic epileptogenicity of the FCD II type dysgenetic lesions is related to a complex histopathophysiology. According to the review of Abdijadid et al. (2015), the dysplastic (dysmorphic, cytomegalic, and immature) neurons are the essential pathogenic elements, unlike the balloon cells, which are not epileptogenic. The cytomegalic interneurons are highly hyperexcitable and display spontaneous membrane depolarizations similar to depolarization shifts. There was an abnormal N-methyl-D-aspartate (NMDA) receptor distribution as well. 4-Aminopyridine-induced ictal discharges were abolished by the NMDA antagonists. The studied tissues showed abnormal GABA receptor–mediated epileptiform field potentials and overlapping ictal discharges. The cytomegalic and immature pyramidal neurons worked predominantly with GABAergic synaptic activity. Surprisingly, GABA acts here as an excitatory transmitter not responding to benzodiazepines. The abnormal GABA activity shows intradysplastic self-sustained pacemaker-like activity, producing continuous and rhythmic epileptiform discharges. The expression of the GABAergic interneurons is low and the calbindin- and parvalbumin-containing cells distribute abnormally. The mechanistic target of rapamycin pathway shows dysfunctional features as well.

We conclude that an important group of the lesional sleep-related frontal lobe epilepsies is related to a histologically homogeneous dysplastic lesion, Taylor type IIb FCD. Robust epileptogenic seizure-prone interictal/semiictal EEG features as well as an excellent postresection outcome of the underlying FCD characterize this group. It seems obvious that although the seizure semiology is roughly similar to that of NFLEs in general, this group makes a distinct entity with a clear etiology, strong intrinsic epileptogenicity, and good surgical treatability. Although it demands more interventions than the rest of the epilepsies, there is a better prospect for a complete recovery. Although the epilepsy of the idiopathic/cryptogenic group is less dramatic, the chance for their complete recovery falls behind. Further analysis of the seizure symptoms in the FCD type II group will shed more light on the seizure types in the sleep-related frontal epilepsy group.

We need to note that mainly the functional–anatomical relations, regardless of the etiology, shape the specific seizure symptoms, whereas sleep relatedness is caused by the highly epileptogenic histology type. The tissue of FCD II produces abundant spikes during sleep, determining sleep relatedness. Another aspect needs some more reflection. Apart from a few ADNFLE families manifesting mental deficits (Picard et al., 2009), there is astonishingly little neuropsychological loss in NFLE. The effects of intensive and continuous spiking during the SWS in the FCD group might forecast a cognitive decay; however, this question needs further study. It is likely that there is more cognitive impairment than detected by now, remaining hidden either because of the few studies devoted to this field or because the functional deficits of these frontal lobe–affected patients mainly impair their socioeconomical and personality traits rather than the traditional neuropsychological parameters (Helmstaedter, 2001)

The complex interrelationship of the aspects determining sleep-related frontal lobe epilepsies with or without a lesion can be summarized as follows.

There are seizures of variable complexity, from seemingly plain arousals, through movements related to the frontostriatal motor network, to behavioral and autonomic signs of alarm and panic with hypermotor movement storms. There is partial evidence for the relationship between the anatomical site of seizure onset (within the frontal lobe) and the semiology of symptoms, independent of the histological type of the lesions.

Of all the lesional cases, FCD type II has the strongest sleep relatedness both for seizures and for interictal spiking. The seizure semiological spectrum of lesional and nonlesional (with or without gene mutations) seems not to differ much; however, this comparison has not been statistically analyzed yet.

SUMMARY OF ABSENCE EPILEPSY AND NOCTURNAL FRONTAL LOBE EPILEPSY CHAPTERS

1. Experimental research has proven that the spike-wake pattern of absence epilepsy and the NREM sleep-related burst-firing mode of the cortico-thalamic system share the same functional structures in the brain. Clinical research has shown that absences occur when the vigilance decreases, during transitions from waking to NREM sleep; whereas wakefulness and REM sleep inhibit them. Those sensory stimuli, which elicit slow wave responses during the transition states (reactive slow waves, i.e. CAP A1 phase), may activate spike wave responses, while those eliciting desynchronization-arousal responses, may not.

   Therefore, in terms of states and functions, absence epilepsy seems to be linked to the periods of initiation and shifts towards NREM sleep.

2. ADNFLE, the genetic variation of NFLE is underlain by mutations of the nicotinic acetylcholine receptor -system. The Ach receptor gene mutations render the cholinergic ascending arousal system over-sensitive to arousals during NREM sleep; resulting in arousal-linked seizure fragments and full-blown seizures with behavioural manifestations; from plain arousal behaviours to alarm reactions with hypermotor features. The semiology and the occurrence-pattern of seizures can be explained by an increased propensity to arousal and a dissociation between the partially activated brain and a sleeping (dysfunctional) dorso-frontal cortical system. The clinical semiology of the genetic variations and sporadic cases do not differ.

   Therefore, ADNFL and NFLE seems to be linked with the epileptically facilitated cholinergic arousal system; underlain by a genetic or a suspected genetic origin.

   Arousal parasomnias manifest similar but non-epileptic- behaviours as NFLE. The two (epileptic and non-epileptic) conditions show a family clustering with cumulated and mixed cases of both conditions in families or individuals; and probably share the pathomechanism related to dissociative features.

   NFLE and AP (the epileptic and non-epileptic counterparts) may both be linked to a disorder of the frontal part of the ascending arousal system.

3. Based upon the above concepts we propose that AE and NFLE, both idiopathic major thalamo-frontal epilepsies; are system-epilepsies; taking place in the physiological antagonistic twin sleep/arousal network. (Fig. 3.1) The concept of reflex epilepsies is extended here beyond the classical sensory reflex epilepsies to such epilepsies which

are induced by the activation of certain epileptically facilitated brain functions as sleep or arousal.

In absence epilepsy, the ictal activation (absences) occurs during transitional states from wakefulness to sleep while the interictal discharges emerge in deeper sleep stages. In contrast to other sleep related epilepsies, the sleep activation does not seem to result in cognitive decline, possibly because the interictal activation is not so excessive.

In NFLE the arousal presents in a distorted and augmented form (variable severity seizures with arousal and alarm several times during a night); however, both ictal and interictal epileptic EEG activity is weak.

References

Abdijadid, S., Mathern, G.W., Levine, M.S., Cepeda, C., 2015. Basic mechanisms of epileptogenesis in pediatric cortical dysplasia. CNS Neurosci. Ther. 21 (2), 92–103.

Bassetti, C., Vella, S., Donati, F., Wielepp, P., Weder, B., 2000. SPECT during sleepwalking. Lancet 356 (9228), 484–485.

Bisulli, F., Vignatelli, L., Naldi, I., Licchetta, L., Provini, F., Plazzi, G., Di Vito, L., Ferioli, S., Montagna, P., Tinuper, P., 2010. Increased frequency of arousal parasomnias in families with nocturnal frontal lobe epilepsy: a common mechanism? Epilepsia 51 (9), 1852–1860.

Broughton, R.J., 1968. Sleep disorders: disorders of arousal? Enuresis, somnambulism, and nightmares occur in confusional states of arousal, not in "dreaming sleep". Science 159 (3819), 1070–1078.

Carrera, E., Tononi, G., 2014. Diaschisis: past, present, future. Brain 137 (Pt. 9), 2408–2422.

Chen, Z., Wang, L., Wang, C., Chen, Q., Zhai, Q., Guo, Y., Zhang, Y., 2015. Mutational analysis of CHRNB2, CHRNA2 and CHRNA4 genes in Chinese population with autosomal dominant nocturnal frontal lobe epilepsy. Int. J. Clin. Exp. Med. 8 (6), 9063–9070.

Cordeiro, M.I., von Ellenrieder, N., Zazubovits, N., Dubeau, F., Gotman, J., Frauscher, B., 2015. Sleep influences the intracerebral EEG pattern of focal cortical dysplasia. Epilepsy Res. 113, 132–139.

Derry, C.P., Davey, M., Johns, M., Kron, K., Glencross, D., Marini, C., Scheffer, I.E., Berkovic, S.F., 2006. Distinguishing sleep disorders from seizures: diagnosing bumps in the night. Arch. Neurol. 63 (5), 705–709.

Derry, C.P., Harvey, A.S., Walker, M.C., Duncan, J.S., Berkovic, S.F., 2009. NREM arousal parasomnias and their distinction from nocturnal frontal lobe epilepsy: a video EEG analysis. Sleep 32 (12), 1637–1644.

Descarries, L., Gisiger, V., Steriade, M., 1997. Diffuse transmission by acetylcholine in the CNS. Prog. Neurobiol. 53 (5), 603–625.

Ebner, A., Dinner, D.S., Noachtar, S., Luders, H., 1995. Automatisms with preserved responsiveness: a lateralizing sign in psychomotor seizures. Neurology 45 (1), 61–64.

Englot, D.J., Yang, L., Hamid, H., Danielson, N., Blumenfeld, H., et al., 2010. Impaired consciousness in temporal lobe seizures: role of cortical slow activity. Brain 133 (Pt. 12), 3764–3777.

Giber, K., Diana, M.A., Plattner, V.M., Dugué, G.P., Acsády, L., 2015. A subcortical inhibitory signal for behavioral arrest in the thalamus. Nat. Neurosci. 18 (4), 562–568.

Halász, P., Bódizs, R., 2013. Dynamic Structure of NREM Sleep. Springer, Berlin, Germany.

Halász, P., Terzano, M., Parrino, L., Bódizs, R., 2004. The nature of arousal in sleep. J. Sleep. Res. 13 (1), 1–23.

Halász, P., Kelemen, A., Szucs, A., 2012. Physiopathogenetic interrelationship between nocturnal frontal lobe epilepsy and NREM arousal parasomnias. Epilepsy Res. Trea 2012, 312693.

Halász, P., Kelemen, A., Szucs, A., 2013. The role of NREM sleep micro-arousals in absence epilepsy and in nocturnal frontal lobe epilepsy. Epilepsy Res. 107 (1–2), 9–19.

Han, Z.Y., Le Novère, N., Zoli, M., Hill Jr., J.A., Champtiaux, N., Changeux, J.P., 2000. Localization of nAChR subunit mRNAs in the brain of Macaca mulatta. Eur. J. Neurosci. 12 (10), 3664–3674.

Haun, F., Eckenrode, T.C., Murray, M., August 1992. Habenula and thalamus cell transplants restore normal sleep behaviors disrupted by denervation of the interpeduncular nucleus. J. Neurosci. 12 (8), 3282–3290.

Helmstaedter, C., 2001. Behavioral aspects of frontal lobe epilepsy. Epilepsy Behav. 2 (5), 384–395.

Hildebrand, M.S., Tankard, R., Gazina, E.V., Damiano, J.A., Lawrence, K.M., Dahl, H.H., Regan, B.M., Shearer, A.E., Smith, R.J., Marini, C., Guerrini, R., Labate, A., Gambardella, A., Tinuper, P., Lichetta, L., Baldassari, S., Bisulli, F., Pippucci, T., Scheffer, I.E., Reid, C.A., Petrou, S., Bahlo, M., Berkovic, S.F., 2015. PRIMA1 mutation: a new cause of nocturnal frontal lobe epilepsy. Ann. Clin. Transl. Neurol. 2 (8), 821–830.

Itier, V., Bertrand, D., 2002. Mutations of the neuronal nicotinic acetylcholine receptors and their association with ADNFLE. Neurophysiol. Clin. 32 (2), 99–107.

Kattler, H., Dijk, D.J., Borbély, A.A., 1994. Effect of unilateral somatosensory stimulation prior to sleep on the sleep EEG in humans. J. Sleep. Res. 3 (3), 159–164.

Krueger, J.M., Obál Jr., F., Kapás, L., Fang, J., 1995. Brain organization and sleep function. Behav. Brain Res. 69 (1–2), 177–185.

Kurahashi, H., Hirose, S., May 16, 2002. Autosomal dominant nocturnal frontal lobe epilepsy (updated 2015 Feb 19). In: GeneReviews® [Internet]. University of Washington, Seattle (WA).

Léna, C., Popa, D., Grailhe, R., Escourrou, P., Changeux, J.-P., Adrien, J., 2004. β2-containing nicotinic receptors contribute to the organization of sleep and regulate putative micro-arousals in mice. J. Neurosci. 24 (25), 5711–5718.

Liu, H., Lu, C., Li, Z., Zhou, S., Li, X., Ji, L., Lu, Q., Lv, R., Wu, L., Ma, X., 2011. The identification of a novel mutation of nicotinic acetylcholine receptor gene CHRNB2 in a Chinese patient:iIts possible implication in non-familial nocturnal frontal lobe epilepsy. Epilepsy Res. 95 (1–2), 94–99.

Llinas, R.R., 2002. Fixed action patterns: automatic brain modules that make complex movements. In: Llinás, R.R. (Ed.), I of the Vortex: From Neurons to Self. MIT press, London, UKl, pp. 133–153.

Lugaresi, E., Cirignotta, F., Montagna, P., 1986. Nocturnal paroxysmal dystonia. J. Neurol. Neurosurg. Psychiatry 49 (4), 375–380.

Lyamin, O.I., Manger, P.R., Ridgway, S.H., Mukhametov, L.M., 2008. Siegel JM.Cetacean sleep: an unusual form of mammalian sleep. Neurosci. Biobehav. Rev. 32 (8), 1451–1484.

Mahowald, M.W., 2002. Arousal and sleep-wake transition parasomnias. In: Lee-Chiong, T.J., Sateia, M.J., Carskadon, M.A. (Eds.), SleepMedicine. Hanley and Belfus, Philadelphia, PA, USA, pp. 207–213.

Mahowald, M.W., Schenk, C.H., 1992. Dissociated states of wakefulness and sleep. Neurology 42 (7 Suppl 6), 44–51.

Manford, M., Fish, D.R., Shorvon, S.D., 1996. An analysis of clinical seizure patterns and their localizing value in frontal and temporal lobe epilepsies. Brain 119 (Pt. 1), 17–40.

Montagna, P., Provini, F., Bisulli, F., Tinuper, P., 2008. Nocturnal epileptic seizures versus the arousal parasomnias. Somnologie 12, 25–37.

Morris 3rd, H.H., Dinner, D.S., Lüders, H., Wyllie, E., Kramer, R., 1988. Supplementary motor seizures: clinical and electroencephalographic findings. Neurology 38 (7), 1075–1082.

Mukhametov, L.M., Supin, A.Y., Polyakova, I.G., 1977. Interhemispheric asymmetry of the electroencephalographic sleep patterns in dolphins. Brain Res. 134 (3), 581–584.

Muzur, A., Pace-Schott, .E.F., Hobson, J.A., 2002. The prefrontal cortex in sleep. Trends Cogn. Sci. 6, 475–481.

Nobili, L., Cardinale, F., Magliola, U., Cicolin, A., Didato, G., Bramerio, M., Fuschillo, D., Spreafico, R., Mai, R., Sartori, I., Francione, S., Lo Russo, G., Castana, L., Tassi, L., Cossu, M., 2009. Taylor's focal cortical dysplasia increases the risk of sleep-related epilepsy. Epilepsia 50 (12), 2599–2604.

Oldani, A., Zucconi, M., Ferini-Strambi, L., Bizzozero, D., Smirne, S., 1996. Autosomal dominant nocturnal frontal lobe epilepsy: electroclinical picture. Epilepsia 37 (10), 964–976.

Palmini, A., Gambardella, A., Andermann, F., Dubeau, F., da Costa, J.C., Olivier, A., Tampieri, D., Gloor, P., Quesney, F., Andermann, E., et al., 1995. Intrinsic epileptogenicity of human dysplastic cortex as suggested by corticography and surgical results. Ann. Neurol. 37 (4), 476–487.

Parrino, L., De Paolis, F., Milioli, G., Gioi, G., Grassi, A., Riccardi, S., Colizzi, E., Terzano, M., 2012. Sleep fingerprints in nocturnal frontal lobe epilepsy: the impact of homeostatic and arousal mechanisms on ictal events. Epilepsia 53, 1178–1184.

Picard, F., Bruel, D., Servent, D., Saba, W., Fruchart-Gaillard, C., Schollhorn-Peyronneau, M.A., Roumenov, D., Brodtkorb, .E., Zuberi, S., Gambardella, A., Steinborn, B., Hufnagel, A., Valette, H., Bottlaender, M., 2006. Alteration of the in vivo nicotinic receptor density in ADNFLE patients: a PET study. Brain. 129, 2047–2060. https://www.ncbi.nlm.nih.gov/pubmed/9148196.

Picard, F., Pegna, A.J., Arntsberg, V., Lucas, N., Kaczmarek, I., Todica, O., Chiriaco, C., Seeck, M., Brodtkorb, E., 2009. Neuropsychological disturbances in frontal lobe epilepsy due to mutated nicotinic receptors. Epilepsy Behav. 14 (2), 354–359.

Provini, F., Plazzi, G., Tinuper, P., Vandi, S., Lugaresi, E., 1999. Montagna P.Nocturnal frontal lobe epilepsy. A clinical and polygraphic overview of 100 consecutive cases. Brain 122 (Pt. 6), 1017–1031.

Rozycka, A., Skorupska, E., Kostyrko, A., Trzeciak, W.H., 2003. Evidence for S284L mutation of the CHRNA4 in a white family with autosomal dominant nocturnal frontal lobe epilepsy. Epilepsia 44 (8), 1113–1117.

Scheffer, I.E., Bhatia, K.P., Lopes-Cendes, I., Fish, D.R., Marsden, C.D., Andermann, E., Andermann, F., Desbiens, R., Keene, D., Cendes, F., Manson, J.I., Constantinou, J.E.C., McIntosh, A.F., Berkovic, S., 1995. Autosomal dominant nocturnal frontal lobe epilepsy. A distinctive clinical disorder. Brain 118 (Pt. 1), 61–73.

Tassi, L., Garbelli, R., Colombo, N., Bramerio, M., Russo, G.L., Mai, R., Deleo, F., Francione, S., Nobili, L., Spreafico, R., 2012. Electroclinical, MRI and surgical outcomes in 100 epileptic patients with type II FCD. Epileptic Disord. 14 (3), 257–266.

Tassinari, C.A., Rubboli, G., Gardella, E., et al., 2005. Central pattern generators for a common semiology in fronto-limbic seizures and in parasomnias. A neuroethologic approach. Neurol. Sci. 26 (Suppl. 3), s225–s232.

Terzaghi, M., Sartori, I., Tassi, L., Didato, G., Rustioni, V., LoRusso, G., Manni, R., Nobili, L., 2009. Evidence of dissociated arousal states during NREM parasomnia from an intracerebral neurophysiological study. Sleep 32 (3), 409–412.

Tinuper, P., Bisulli, F., Cross, J.H., Hesdorffer, D., Kahane, P., Nobili, L., Provini, F., Scheffer, I.E., Tassi, L., Vignatelli, L., Bassetti, C., Cirignotta, F., Derry, C., Gambardella, A., Guerrini, R., Halasz, P., Licchetta, L., Mahowald, M., Manni, R., Marini, C., Mostacci, B., Naldi, I., Parrino, L., Picard, F., Pugliatti, M., Ryvlin, P., Vigevano, F., Zucconi, M., Berkovic, S., Ottman, R., 2016 10. Definition and diagnostic criteria of sleep-related hypermotor epilepsy. Neurology 86 (19), 1834–1842.

Waterman, K., Purves, S.J., Kosaka, B., 1987. An epileptic syndrome caused by mesial frontal lobe seizure foci. Neurology 37 (4), 577–582.

Weltzin, M.M., Lindstrom, J.M., Lukas, R.J., Whiteaker, P., 2016. Distinctive effects of nicotinic receptor intracellular-loop mutations associated with nocturnal frontal lobe epilepsy. Neuropharmacology 102, 158–173.

Williamson, P.D., Spencer, D.D., Spencer, S.S., Novelly, R.A., Mattson, R.H., 1985. Complex partial seizures of frontal lobe origin. Ann. Neurol. 18 (4), 497–504.

Zucconi, M., Oldani, A., Smirne, S., Ferini-Strambi, L., 2000. The macrostructure and microstructure of sleep in patients with autosomal dominant nocturnal frontal lobe epilepsy. J. Clin. Neurophysiol. 17 (1), 77–86.

Juvenile Idiopathic Myoclonic Epilepsy (Janz Syndrome) as a System Epilepsy Affecting the Corticothalamic System and the Frontal Motor and Cognitive Frontal Subsystems

In 70% of cases, this condition starts after adolescence, between 11 and 20 years of age, or in young adulthood. Antiepileptic drugs, especially valproic acid, make patients permanently seizure-free; however, reducing and stopping medication may result in the recurrence of seizures even after 5 years' freedom from seizures, even in late adulthood.

Some patients are able to stop antiepileptic medications, but there are no features identifying those prone to remaining seizure-free. Höfler et al. (2014) have shown that fewer of the patients having just one seizure type remained seizure-free after stopping medication compared to those patients with variable seizures—absences, myocloni, or generalized tonic–clonic (GTC)—before the successful treatment period.

Juvenile idiopathic myoclonic epilepsy (JME) makes up about 3%–6% of all epilepsies. There are three types of seizures: (1) The first type are myoclonic jerks (singular ones or clusters of arrhythmic, irregular patterns) with no loss of consciousness, typically affecting the extensor muscles of the upper limbs, especially in the morning hours. Massive myocloni may result in falls. The jerks prefer the periods around GTC seizures and they make up the only seizure type in 8%–17% of JME cases. (2) GTC seizures are rare; several years may go without them. (3) Absence seizures occur in 15%–40% of JME cases. Sleep loss and sleep deprivation are strong seizure-provoking factors; the attacks frequently occur during the sleep period after sleep deprivation or at awakening.

The typical EEG symptoms are short, 1- to 3-s, high-voltage polyspike–wave paroxysms not easily captured by routine EEG but by sleep EEG, occurring while falling asleep, typically during awakening, or during a sleep period after awakening. EEG spikes and myocloni do not correlate. The short polyspike and spike–wave bursts of sleep EEG typically associate with the cyclic alternating pattern (CAP) phase A1.

A feature of the syndrome occurring in about 50% of patients is "reflex seizures": attacks evoked by a consistent triggering stimulus. It is likely that a reflex mechanism is a hidden trigger for many apparently "spontaneous" seizures in JME. There are several types of triggering stimuli: photosensitivity, eye closure and eye opening, and different activity (praxis) types, including speech and reading as well, making up the syndrome of reading epilepsy (see the next section). Wolf (2015) described four types of evoking stimuli and reflex epileptic features:

1. Genetic *photosensitivity* is the best-known type (Wolf and Goosses, 1986), in the form of the photoparoxysmal response provoked in up to 90% of JME patients if sufficient light intensity was applied (Appleton et al., 2000). This pathologic response to intermittent flashing light stimulation develops in the occipital region first, and then it spreads bilaterally and anteriorly along the cortex, not affecting the thalamus (Moeller et al., 2009).

2. Sensitivity to eye closure (*fixation off activity*): The closure of the eyes triggers spike–waves immediately. The syndrome affects 15%–20% of JME patients. This type of sensitivity is the leading sign of Jeavons syndrome (eyelid myoclonia with absences), overlapping with photosensitivity.

3. *Orofacial reflex myocloni*: Rapid small jerks in the perioral muscles, in the tongue and chin, activated by language-related activities such as reading and speech. This type of reflex myocloni defines the syndrome of reading epilepsy (Yacubian and Wolf, 2015), affecting 25%–30% of JME patients. It is realized by a widespread, bilateral network associated with speech-related functions. EEG–functional

magnetic resonance imaging (fMRI) investigations have shown that a critical amount of corticoreticular and corticocortical neurons need to activate to reach the stimulus threshold of the network for producing the pathological reflex seizure (Salek-Haddadi et al., 2009).

4. In *praxis-related reflex epilepsy* the myocloni are triggered by complex motor activities, led by cognition. This syndrome affects about half of Japanese and 24%–29% of other JME patients (Matsuoka et al., 2000; Yacubian and Wolf, 2014).

Janz noticed the peculiar *personality traits* of JME patients even at the first description of the condition; however, their full and unequivocal account could be the yield of sophisticated neuropsychological methods linked to modern neuroimaging. Although JME patients have normal intellect, they show poorer socioeconomic performance than do healthy controls in everyday life (Camfield and Camfield, 2009; Wandschneider et al., 2013; Zamarian et al., 2013). Based on study results, they show changes in working memory tasks related to the thalamofrontocentral network, as well as in planning and risk-assessment functions. The degree of poor performance in working memory tests is similar to that of frontal lobe epilepsy patients. Fluorodeoxyglucose-positron emission tomography studies revealed lower glucose uptake during cognitive tasks in the ventral premotor cortex, in the caudate nucleus, and in the dorsolateral frontal cortex compared to controls (Swartz et al., 1996).

The genetic and biological basis of behavioral and lifestyle disturbances is supported by JME's psychiatric comorbidity (Gélisse et al., 2001; Somayajula et al., 2015; Trinka et al., 2006). Certain psychiatric signs like emotional instability, immaturity, poor self-discipline, mood swings, sensation seeking, and consistent frontal MRI changes also suggest a typical personality change associated with JME (de Araujo Filho et al., 2013; Syvertsen et al., 2014; Walsh et al., 2014).

The known triggering role of cognitive stress for myocloni supports the possible link of cognitive changes and the seizure mechanism.

Among the multilateral pathologic changes underlying JME, a basic one is the *system-specific increase* in cortical excitability. In addition to myocloni and polyspike–waves, the increased responsiveness to transcranial magnetic stimulation shows the facilitated state of the primary motor system. The degree of this responsivity follows the seizures' diurnal variation: it is most marked after sleep deprivation and in the morning hours (Manganotti et al., 2006; Badawy et al., 2009). The analysis of polyspike–waves has suggested a frontal and a hemispheric dominance; in other words, a frontal seizure-initiating focus within the myoclonus network (Panzica et al., 2001). The LORETA analysis of functional connectivity (Clemens et al., 2013) performed in interictal and periictal periods has evidenced the increased connectivity of the cingulum, the frontal superior and middle gyrus, and the paracentral region.

Neuroimaging studies have revealed an increased connectivity and hyperexcitability as well as dysgenetic elements in the corticothalamic functions such as frontal cognitive performance and in several subsystems of the centrofrontal motor system. There was an abnormal connectivity between the frontopolar and the prefrontal regions as well as between the motor cortex and the frontoparietal working memory fields in JME patients with normal cognitive performance (Vollmar et al., 2012). Performing fMRI and diffusion tensor imaging (DTI) studies in 29 JME patients and healthy controls, they found an increased structural connectivity between the medial prefrontal and the motor cortex. The DTI and fMRI data were correlated: a stronger structural connectivity was associated with a stronger functional connectivity. There was a low connectivity between the prefrontal and the frontopolar regions; and it was high between the occipital region and the supplementary motor area (Fig. 4.1). These connectivity data link seizure semiology with neurophysiology, neuropsychology, and imaging findings. The findings are consistent with earlier data on microstructural white matter changes in JME (Woermann et al., 1999; Tae et al., 2008).

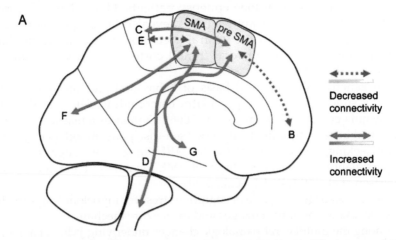

FIGURE 4.1   (A) Summary of the work of Vollmar et al. (2012) with diffusion tensor imaging (DTI). (B) The pre–supplementary motor area (SMA) shows decreased connectivity with the frontopolar region. (C) The connectivity is high between the SMA and the central gyri and between the SMA and the descending motor pathways (D), compared to normal controls. (E) The connectivity is low between the SMA and the central cortical regions; it is high between the occipital (F) and (G) the temporal areas. The functional connectivity measured by EEG–functional MRI between the prefrontal cortex and the SMA was congruent with DTI data. The degree of the SMA connectivity and the severity of clinical symptoms have been positively correlated. These data support an increase in the microstructural connectivity between the motor system and the frontal cognitive system. The increased connectivity with the descending motor pathways may explain the myocloni. The increased connectivity with the occipital areas may explain photoparoxysmal sensitivity. The decreased connectivity of the pre-SMA and the frontopolar cortex is in keeping with the frontal cognitive deficit symptoms. These data well illustrate the possibility of multiple system errors.

By linking connectivity data with the age at seizure onset in JME, a developmental origin of the abnormal connectivity features seems likely. The cortex undergoes important structural changes during adolescence, while the power of sleep slow waves decreases together with the pruning of the cortical synapses. During this vehement developmental process paralleling the first occurrence of JME seizures critical mistakes might occur, leading to JME. Because this sophisticated developmental process is under the control of the fine-tuned cooperation of several regulatory genes, variable genetic changes might influence the development of JME.

Neuroimaging and neuropsychological data have highlighted new features of the syndrome, clarifying old and doubtful strains. It seems that JME cannot be fit into the procrustean bed of "generalized epilepsy," rather, the new strains make it a good muster for system epilepsies (even if too many systems appear to be involved).

Still, one may ask, do those features classifying JME earlier into the idiopathic generalized epilepsy group make a link between absence epilepsy and JME? The endophenotypic features of EEG do certainly represent such a link; however, there are some contradictions in this respect. The generalized spike–wave pattern of absence epilepsy turns to a polyspike–wave variant in JME, activated by superficial sleep, closer to waking than the absences' spike–wave pattern, which is rather linked closer to stage 2 sleep. At the same time, both patterns associate with CAP A1. Absence seizures may represent another overlapping endophenotype with identical fMRI features, EEG, and clinical seizure symptoms. It is likely that both syndromes relate to an identical or very similar dysfunction of the corticothalamic system, but many more subsystems may be involved in JME, for which both clinical and neuroimaging data suggest the participation of motor and cognitive networks. As for age dependency, where absence epilepsy comes to an end, JME starts. This means that the dramatic developmental switch of childhood to adolescence, inhibiting absence epilepsy, permits or rather evokes JME-related dysfunctions.

In the next section, we shall discuss reading epilepsies, showing an important symptomatic overlap with JME, making the two conditions suspected to be parts of one spectrum disorder.

READING EPILEPSY: A RELATED SYNDROME

Although Bickford described reading epilepsy as early as 1956, this type of epilepsy has hardly been known, because of its rarity and being under-investigated. It is not its practical importance, but rather its heuristic significance that makes it worth dealing with this condition now. Its heuristic significance relates to being the epilepsy of a sophisticated, highly organized cognitive system. It is "system epilepsy"; the seizures are induced by specific activities such as reading, speech, and—rarely—thinking, whereas spontaneous attacks hardly occur. It is usually recognized in adolescence (11–22 years, median 15 years).

The two forms of reading epilepsy are the following (Koutroumanidis et al., 1998):

1. In the common variant, reading triggers orofacial (chin) jerks. Generally, there is no disturbance of consciousness, just a momentary thinking block, "dizziness," or "losing the thread of conversation." The ictal EEG is characterized by short spike–waves or sharp–slow waves and occasional singular slow waves. The jerks and EEG discharges are not always synchronous. Some discharges are bilateral, frontal, and more prominent on the dominant side.
2. The rare variant is not associated with myocloni, but rather to dysphasic episodes with discomfort and a mild dizziness, evoked by reading. The ictal EEG consists of prolonged focal/regional dominant-side posterior temporoparietooccipital slow and sharp wave runs.

The condition has a genetic background. Family patterns such as parent–child, identical twin pair, and nonsymptomatic spike–wave pattern evoked by reading in first-degree relatives, as well as the presence of other hereditary epilepsy types in the patient's family have been described. There is a possible link between reading epilepsy and JME, not systematically investigated.

Neuroimaging studies have identified potentially responsible hyperexcitable networks for the syndrome: a circumscribed area in the dominant angular gyrus region in the posterior temporal variant and a bitemporo/bifrontal network in the myoclonus variant (Salek-Haddadi et al., 2009). FMRI studies have shown blood oxygen level–dependent (BOLD) activation during reading-induced myocloni in the dominant motor and premotor cortices as well as in the striate nucleus, the mesiotemporal limbic area, the Brodmann area, and the thalamus. The activation overlapped the neighboring regions covering the area of physiologic speech activation. Vaudano et al. (2012) performed an fMRI series in a reading epilepsy patient. At the onset of myocloni, the BOLD activation first appeared in the deep pyriformis cortex and in the Brodmann area, then in the thalamus and the subdominant lower frontal region. The Brodmann area proved to be the link between cognitive activation and seizures. Reading, the common evoking stimulus, transforms the linguistic "raw material" to speech.

The hyperexcitability of the speech network underlies reading epilepsy. If the speech network is activated by reading or any verbal activity, it is prone to producing a seizure. We can catch in action a sophisticated, multilateral cognitive function turning into epileptic activity underlain by the hyperexcitability of the system.

CLASSIFICATION ISSUES AND CONTROVERSIES BETWEEN THE GENETIC, ELECTROENCEPHALOGRAPHIC, COGNITIVE, AND MOTOR FEATURES OF JME AND READING EPILEPSY

Several novel features of JME and reading epilepsy have been discovered since the 1990s. JME has seceded from the idiopathic generalized epilepsy group, which is not a tenable construction any more. At the same time, however, the relation of JME with sleep (the epileptic sensitivity to sleep deprivation) has remained an essential feature. The bilateral synchronous short polyspike–wave paroxysms associate with CAP phase A1, especially with the reactive slow waves of sleep (Gigli et al., 1992), similar to absence-type spike–wave discharge. The newly recognized reflex features of JME shed new light on its link with reading epilepsy. The data on frontal cognitive symptoms and the presence of motor network abnormalities in JME support its frontal lobe relations.

The multilevel incongruence regarding the EEG, seizure semiology, and genotypic features of JME obstructs its clear classification. Time is not yet ripe to combine the seemingly incongruent elements into a new construction. We discuss this delicate part of epileptology to demonstrate the need for change in our syndrome classifications reflecting the actual trends and concepts.

References

Appleton, R., Beirne, M., Acomb, B., 2000. Photosensitivity in juvenile myoclonic epilepsy. Seizure 9 (2), 108–111.

Badawy, R.A., Macdonell, R.A., Jackson, G.D., Berkovic, S.F., 2009. Why do seizures in generalized epilepsy often occur in the morning? Neurology 73 (3), 218–222.

Camfield, C.S., Camfield, P.R., September 29, 2009. Juvenile myoclonic epilepsy 25 years after seizure onset: a population-based study. Neurology 73 (13), 1041–1045.

Clemens, B., Puskás, S., Besenyei, M., Spisák, T., Opposits, G., Hollódy, K., Fogarasi, A., Fekete, I., Emri, M., 2013. Neurophysiology of juvenile myoclonic epilepsy: EEG-based network and graph analysis of the interictal and immediate preictal states. Epilepsy Res. 106 (3), 357–369.

de Araujo Filho, G.M., de Araujo, T.B., Sato, J.R., Silva, I., Lin, K., Júnior, H.C., Yacubian, E.M., Jackowski, A.P., 2013. Personality traits in juvenile myoclonic epilepsy: evidence of cortical abnormalities from a surface morphometry study. Epilepsy Behav. 27 (2), 385–392.

Gélisse, P., Genton, P., Samuelian, J.C., Thomas, P., Bureau, M., 2001. Psychiatric disorders in juvenile myoclonic epilepsy. Rev. Neurol. (Paris) 157 (3), 297–302.

Gigli, G.L., Calia, E., Narciani, M.G., Mazza, S., Mennuni, G., Diomedi, M., Terzano, M.G., Janz, D., 1992. Sleep microstructure and EEG epileptiform activity in patients with juvenile myoclonic epilepsy. Epilepsia 33 (5), 799–804.

Höfler, J., Unterberger, I., Dobesberger, J., Kuchukhidze, G., Walser, G., Trinka, E., 2014. Seizure outcome in 175 patients with juvenile myoclonic epilepsy-a long-term observational study. Epilepsy Res. 108 (10), 1817–1824.

Koutroumanidis, M., Koepp, M.J., Richardson, M.P., Camfield, C., Agathonikou, A., Ried, S., Papadimitriou, A., Plant, G.T., Duncan, J.S., Panayiotopoulos, C.P., Agathonikou, A., et al., 1998. The variants of reading epilepsy. A clinical and video-EEG study of 17 patients with reading-induced seizures. Brain 121 (Pt 8), 1409–1427.

Manganotti, P., Bongiovanni, L.G., Fuggetta, G., Zanette, G., Fiaschi, A., 2006. Effects of sleep deprivation on cortical excitability in patients affected by juvenile myoclonic epilepsy: a combined transcranial magnetic stimulation and EEG study. J. Neurol. Neurosurg. Psychiatry 77 (1), 56–60.

Matsuoka, H.1, Takahashi, T., Sasaki, M., Matsumoto, K., Yoshida, S., Numachi, Y., Saito, H., Ueno, T., 2000. Brain 123 (Pt 2), 318–330.

Moeller, F., Siebner, H.R., Ahlgrimm, N., Wolff, S., Muhle, H., et al., 2009. fMRI activation during spike and wave discharges evoked by photic stimulation. Neuroimage 48 (4), 682–695.

Panzica, F., Rubboli, G., Franceschetti, S., Avanzini, G., Meletti, S., Pozzi, A., Tassinari, C.A., 2001. Cortical myoclonus in Janz syndrome. Clin. Neurophysiol. 112 (10), 1803–1809.

Salek-Haddadi, A., Mayer, T., Hamandi, K., Symms, M., Josephs, O., Fluegel, D., Woermann, F., Richardson, M.P., Noppeney, U., Wolf, P., Koepp, M.J., 2009. Imaging seizure activity: a combined EEG/EMG-fMRI study in reading epilepsy. Epilepsia 50 (2), 256–264.

Somayajula, S., Vooturi, S., Jayalakshmi, S., 2015. Psychiatric disorders among 165 patients with juvenile myoclonic epilepsy in India and association with clinical and sociodemographic variables. Epilepsy Behav. 53, 37–42.

Swartz, B.E., Simpkins, F., Halgren, E., Mandelkern, M., Brown, C., Krisdakumtorn, T., Gee, M., 1996. Visual working memory in primary generalized epilepsy: an 18FDG-PET study. Neurology 47 (5), 1203–1212.

Syvertsen, M.R., Thuve, S., Stordrange, B.S., Brodtkorb, E., 2014. Clinical heterogeneity of juvenile myoclonic epilepsy: follow-up after an interval of more than 20 years. Seizure 23 (5), 344–348.

Tae, W.S., Kim, S.H., Joo, E.Y., Han, S.J., Kim, I.Y., Kim, S.I., Lee, J.M., Hong, S.B., 2008. Cortical thickness abnormality in juvenile myoclonic epilepsy. J. Neurol. 255 (4), 561–566.

Trinka, E., Kienpointner, G., Unterberger, I., Luef, G., Bauer, G., Doering, L.B., Doering, S., 2006. Psychiatric comorbidity in juvenile myoclonic epilepsy. Epilepsia 47 (12), 2086–2091.

Vaudano, A.E., Carmichael, D.W., Salek-Haddadi, A., Rampp, S., Stefan, H., Lemieux, L., Koepp, M., 2012. Networks involved in seizure initiation. A reading epilepsy case studied with EEG-fMRI and MEG. J. Neurol. 79 (3), 249–253.

Vollmar, C., O'Muircheartaigh, J., Symms, M.R., Barker, G.J., Thompson, P., Kumari, V., Stretton, J., Duncan, J.S., Richardson, M.P., Koepp, M.J., 2012. Altered microstructural connectivity in juvenile myoclonic epilepsy: the missing link. Neurology 78 (20), 15.

Walsh, J., Thomas, R.H., Church, C., Rees, M.I., Marson, A.G., et al., 2014. Executive functions and psychiatric symptoms in drug-refractory juvenile myoclonic epilepsy. Epilepsy Behav. 35, 72–77.

Wandschneider, B., Centeno, M., Vollmar, C., Stretton, J., O'Muircheartaigh, J., Thompson, P.J., Kumari, V., Symms, M., Barker, G.J., Duncan, J.S., Richardson, M.P., Koepp, M.J., 2013. Risk-taking behavior in juvenile myoclonic epilepsy. Epilepsia 54 (12), 2158–2165.

Woermann, F.G., Free, S.L., Koepp, M.J., Sisodiya, S.M., Duncan, J.S., 1999. Abnormal cerebral structure in juvenile myoclonic epilepsy demonstrated with voxel-based analysis of MRI. Brain 122 (Pt 11), 2101–2108.

Wolf, P., Goosses, R., 1986. Relation of photosensitivity to epileptic syndromes. J. Neurol. Neurosurg. Psychiatry 49 (12), 1386–1391.

Wolf, P., 2015. Reflex epileptic mechanisms in humans: lessons about natural ictogenesis. Epilepsy Behav. 52 (Pt A), 277–278.

Yacubian, E.M., Wolf, P., 2015. Orofacial reflex myocloni. Definition, relation to epilepsy syndromes, nosological and prognosis significance. A focused review. Seizure 30, 1–5.

Yacubian, E.M., Wolf, P., 2014. Praxis induction, definition, relation to epilepsy syndromes, nosological and prognostic significance, a focused review. Seizure 23 (4), 247–251.

Zamarian, L., Höfler, J., Kuchukhidze, G., Delazer, N., Bonatti, E., Kemmeler, G., Trinka, E., 2013. Decision making in juvenile myoclonic epilepsy. J. Neurol. 260 (3), 839–846.

Medial Temporal Lobe Epilepsy (MTLE): The Epilepsy of the Hippocampal Declarative Memory System

Sleep, Epilepsies, and Cognitive Impairment
http://dx.doi.org/10.1016/B978-0-12-812579-3.00005-4

Because medial temporal lobe epilepsy (MTLE) is the most frequent type of epilepsy, there is great amount of knowledge about its symptoms and mechanisms. Therefore, our endeavor to reinterpret this type of epilepsy might seem surprising. We will discuss three main aspects: (1) the interrelationship of MTLE and memory in the light of new neurophysiology data on declarative (hippocampal) memory consolidation, rendering MTLE the epilepsy of the limbic memory system; (2) the bilateral involvement of the temporal lobes (parts of the limbic system) in MTLE, confirming its system-related, rather than focal/regional, character; and (3) the overall integrative role of slow-wave sleep (SWS).

THE MEMORY PROCESS AND THE ROLE OF THE SHARP WAVE–RIPPLE IN MEMORY ENCODING AND CONSOLIDATION

The memory process involves three steps: encoding, consolidation, and recall. Since the end of the 20th century, increasing evidence has shown that the engrams first develop in a transitory and vulnerable form in the hippocampus (Buzsáki, 2015). They gain a more stable form later, during the consolidation process, contacting other engrams preserved in the frontal cortical stores. This process takes place without conscious awareness, during SWS. The sleep relatedness is not so curious if we take into account that the immediate workup, transmission, and storage of too many data during the daytime would overload the same restricted capacities, not allowing the elaboration of information. The restricted input and the lack of conscious workup during sleep secure better circumstances for the process.

Studies on the effects of sleep on learning have highlighted an increase in both declarative and procedural tasks when the experimental learning was followed by SWS within 16 h. The material consolidated by sleep became more resistant against interference and forgetting (Stickgold and Walker, 2013; Buzsáki, 2015; Feld and Diekelmann, 2015). Chrobak and Buzsáki (1996, 1998), Buzsáki (2015), Born et al. (2006), and Born (2010) explored this second step of the memory process, consolidation, at the turn of the century. These researchers had first assumed, and later they confirmed (Wilson and McNaughton, 1994), a peculiar mechanism for the reactivation (repetition) of memories for strengthening—consolidating—them. After the memory engrams are encoded in the hippocampus during wakefulness, they would be reactivated at a faster speed (like an accelerated film) and in a more condensed form in the same hippocampus, guided by sleep slow oscillation. Then they would be transferred to the frontal neocortex in a consolidated form, joining the stored memories there. This scenario has been confirmed for explicit (declarative) memories, whereas the organization of procedural memories was suggested to be processed by the basal ganglia.

Chemical effects also control the memory process. The hippocampal structure is under the influence of the acetylcholinergic transmitter system. Cholinergic agonists facilitate encoding, whereas they inhibit consolidation, during SWS (Hasselmo, 2006).

A hippocampal electrophysiological pattern having an important impact on memory processing both in experimental animals and in humans has attracted considerable attention: it is the sharp wave–ripple (SPW-r) complex.

The SPW-r is a robust, far-reaching cell-population episode, the most synchronized event of the mammalian brain (Buzsáki, 2015), which augments the excitability of the hippocampus and the connected structures (Buzsáki, 1986; Chrobak, Buzsáki, 1996; Csicsvari et al., 1999). It can elicit long-term potentiation,[1] changing the synaptic weights between hippocampal neurons.

---

[1] Long-term potentiation (LTP) was discovered by Terje Lomo in rabbit hippocampus, in 1966. He stimulated the perforating track of the hippocampus—proceeding to the dentatus of the hippocampus— and registered the response (EPSP). If he applied a serial stimulation, the subsequent stimulus evoked a longer lasting and higher voltage EPSP and the elevated responsivity was permanent (lasted longer). The forerunner of LTP was Donald Hebb, processing the idea of Ramon y Cajal published in as early as 1894. Cajal's theory suggested that the basis of memory was the plasticity of neuronal communication (Brown et al., 1988). He supposed that, in the course of repeat stimulation, the presynaptic neuron induces some kind of growth and metabolic changes in the postsynaptic neuron. The physical and biological bases of this phenomenon have yet been unclear. LTP is associated to the increase of the number of postsynaptic receptors and synaptic transmitters, resulting in a stronger connection of the two cells.

It appears when the hippocampus is released from inhibition during consummatory behavior in waking or in SWS; and it is suppressed in active waking (theta activity in rats). It is the inner event of the hippocampus, detectable in isolated hippocampal slides as well. The "ripple" is a high-frequency event (200 Hz in animals, 150 Hz in humans) originating in the CA1 region of the hippocampal pyramidal layer in close relation to the sharp wave, originating in the CA3 region (Fig. 5.1) (Buzsáki, 1986). The sharp wave is a 40- to 150-ms maximum 2.5-mV amplitude depolarization discharge involving the hippocampal pyramidal cells. Almost half of the hippocampal neurons (50,000–150,000 neurons) participate in it. The ripple is a fast oscillatory response to the sharp wave, a local event between the CA3 pyramidal cells and the perisomatic inhibitory neurons (Schlingloff et al., 2014; Gulyás and Freund, 2015).

Buzsáki (1986) and Chrobak and Buzsáki (1996) worked out a two-step model for the formation and consolidation of memory in rodents. The first

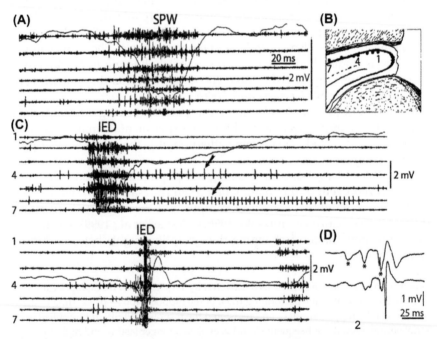

FIGURE 5.1 Sharp wave–ripple (*SPW-r*) and interictal epileptic discharges (*IED*) in rat: laminar unit discharges and field potentials. (A) Neuronal synchrony along the longitudinal axis of the CA1 pyramidal layer during a SPW-r burst in an intact animal. (B) Hippocampus disconnected from its subcortical connections: (C) IEDs appear with afterdischarges (*arrows*) and (D) with greater synchrony and faster and higher amplitude of the field potentials. The figure clearly shows that differences between SPW-r and IEDs are limited.

step is the development of unstable vulnerable hippocampal engrams encoded during the waking theta state, when the afferent activity transitorily changes the synaptic weights through the entorhinal cortex in the CA3 hippocampal region.

The second step occurs during consummatory periods and especially during SWS, when recurrent spontaneous SPW-r events develop owing to the iterative potentiation of the same synapses in which the engram originated during the waking state; the engrams are transferred to the frontal neocortex.

During the reactivation process, the single memory representations (engrams) lose their context-dependent individual features and consolidate in the frontal neocortex like common schema-like extracts (gists) through an "averaging" process. The term "abstraction" refers to the process in which the engrams lose their context-dependent nature during consolidation. The neurophysiological process underlying these changes might involve overlapping fields during iterative reactivations following the Hebbian rules, strengthening the synaptic weights and, consequently, the abstract meanings.

Several studies support the two-step model of memory processing (see Buzsaki's 2015 summary). The "resection" of the SPW ripple episodes provided convincing evidence: no memory consolidation occurred after (Girardeau et al., 2009). Those studies showing that the cellular spike sequences in SWS are identical with the sequences of them during SPW-r events—just faster, compressed in time—have helped the understanding of the consolidation process (Ji and Wilson, 2007; Foster and Wilson, 2006; Nádasdy, 2000). This process could not yet been proven in humans; but the increase in SPW-r episodes after learning seems to be supporting (O'Neill et al., 2008; Cheng and Frank, 2008).

The two-step model was a great step in development. It provided a substrate for memory organization within the temporal lobe and offered a clear neurophysiological mechanism for the encoding and consolidation of memory involving hippocampal and extrahippocampal neocortical structures. At the same time, it explained the clinical experiences of memory disturbances in temporal lobe epilepsy.

Beyond the hippocampo–cortical dialogue, thalamocortical oscillations contribute to the memory process as well (Fig. 5.2). The up states of the slow oscillation ($\leq 1\,Hz$) envelop sleep spindles; and sleep spindles couple with ripples during the learning process (Clemens et al., 2011). The coupling and fine-tuning of these three oscillations render the cortex receptive to plastic changes and orchestrate the hippocampo–cortical dialogue (Born et al., 2006; Born, 2010; Mölle and Born, 2011). The increase in spindle density and the length of stage 2

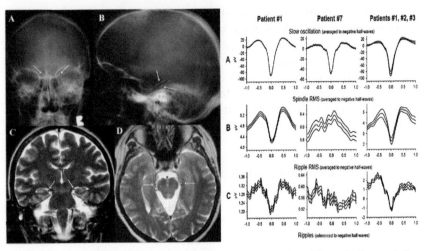

FIGURE 5.2 Temporal coupling of parahippocampal ripples, sleep spindles, and slow oscillations in humans. Left: (A and B) *Arrows* show the locations of the foramen ovale electrodes on the X-ray. (C and D) *Arrows* indicate the MRI at the ambient cistern beside the parahippocampal gyri. Right: Coupling between slow waves (A), spindles (B), and ripples (C) in different patients with medial temporal lobe epilepsy (columns). In columns (1) and (3), in patients with intact hippocampus, the coupling between slow waves and spindles and ripples is shown. The middle column (2) shows that the patient had hippocampal sclerosis. The synchrony in coupling is distorted. *RMS*, Root mean square. *Based on the work of Clemens, Z., Mölle, M., Eross, L., Barsi, P., Halász, P., Born, J., 2007. Temporal coupling of parahippocampal ripples, sleep spindles and slow oscillations in humans. Brain 130 (Pt 11), 2868–2878; with permission.*

SWS during learning show the role of sleep spindling in both visuospatial and verbal memories (Staresina et al., 2015; Fogel and Smith, 2011; Siapas and Wilson, 1998).

Gais et al. (2002) have shown that the frontal spindling density increases during the first 90 min of sleep after performing an intensive declarative memory task. Schabus et al. (2004) compared those subjects who had increased spindle activity after learning with those without. The increase in spindle activity correlated positively with an increased performance after sleep. These results support the role of spindling in the consolidation of declarative memory.

Ample data evidence the role of spindling also in the protection of memory engrams during the consolidation process (Born, 2010; Diekelmann and Born, 2010; Payne and Kensinger, 2011; Lewis and Durrant, 2011). Several important details of the hippocampo–neocortical dialogue wait for further clarification (Buzsáki, 1996, 1998; Diekelmann and Born, 2010). Originally, the "dialogue" appeared unidirectional but now a bidirectional information flow seems more likely.

HOW DOES THE HIPPOCAMPO–NEOCORTICAL MEMORY PROCESS CHANGE DURING MEDIAL TEMPORAL LOBE EPILEPSY?

We have seen that the most important actor in the hippocampal memory process is the SPW-r complex. It is an intensive synchronous excitatory event at the edge of the shift toward epileptic excitation, explaining why the hippocampus is the most epilepsy-prone structure of the brain. The SPW-r pair is the physiological counterpart of the pathological (epileptic) twin pair: the spike–ripple. The high-frequency ripple activity is now recognized as the most essential marker of epilepsy (Buzsáki, 2015). The epileptic spike differs from the sharp wave of the SPW-r only by its shorter duration and higher voltage. Its duration is 30–150 ms and its amplitude does not exceed 2 mV in rats; although in humans the spike amplitude is higher, it is shorter and more synchronously coupled with ripples (Fig. 5.1). This similarity of the physiological and pathological variants clearly shows how easy a shift to epileptic activity is, and shows that the expression "being hijacked" by epilepsy is false. This expression is based on the idea that there is something like "epilepsy" that is completely different from the physiological activity. In reality, epilepsy is rather a derailment of physiological functioning to pathologic malfunctioning: a highly intensive synchronous excitation. This derailment is always possible whenever and wherever important plastic changes occur.

The literature has vividly discussed the detrimental cognitive effects of interictal discharges. Most studies, however, had serious limitations, targeting only waking activity of non-MTLE patients. The intensive sleep activation of interictal discharges has rarely been investigated in MTLE patients (Clemens et al., 2003).

Shatskikh et al. (2006) elicited large population spikes in the CA1 region of hippocampal pyramidal neurons by stimulation of the ventral commissure. They could detect analogue spikes with the spontaneous ones in the CA1 region. The stimulated animals had serious cognitive deficit symptoms in both spatial and verbal memory tasks. This finding supports the hypothesis that interictal spiking may cause memory loss in temporal lobe epilepsy patients.

Frauscher et al. (2015) studied hippocampal sleep spindling in humans with implanted deep electrodes. The hippocampal spindling decreased proportional with the amount of spiking. They assumed that physiological spindling has transformed to spikes in MTLE in analogy with bilateral spike–wave activity, which is considered the pathological counterpart of spindling in idiopathic generalized epilepsy.

Gelinas et al. (2016) provided elegant experimental evidence for the SPW-r transformation into interictal epileptic discharges (IEDs) in a rat kindling model. They showed that the epileptic IEDs interfere as "dummies" with the temporofrontal memory consolidation process.

If these experimental data hold true, an important proportion of memory disturbances in MTLE originate from the ongoing spiking hidden by night sleep, in addition to the static hippocampal sclerosis factor, further ruining memory (Fig. 5.3). Interictal epileptic spiking contributes more to the memory disturbances in MTLE than we had expected.

A 2017 study (Boly et al., 2017) investigated whether epileptic activity can induce plastic changes revealed by increased slow-wave power during non–rapid eye movement (NREM) sleep. They found that the frequency of spiking during the last hours of wakefulness correlated with the increase in slow-wave power during the subsequent NREM sleep period, the slow waves also displaying abnormal topography with a maximum that was concordant with the localization of the seizure-onset zone. Assuming that synaptic potentiation induced by spike firing of epileptic networks is ineffectual, spiking may impair the patient's cognitive performance (Bower et al., 2015). Furthermore, Boyle's study reports

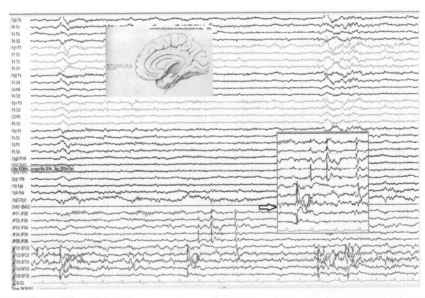

FIGURE 5.3   Sleep recording of a patient with bilateral medial temporal lobe epilepsy performed with foramen ovale (FO) electrodes (top inset: placement of the FO electrodes). The last 10 channels show the records of the FO electrodes: upper 5 channels right side, lower 5 left side. Lower inset: bilateral independent spiking enlarged. There are sleep spindles in the right FO records, no sleep spindles in the left. Abundant interictal spiking is seen continually on both sides, connected with fast activity mainly on the left (congruent with the seizure-onset zone).

also that nighttime interictal spikes are associated with decreased sleep slow-wave homeostasis. This would reduce the physiological synaptic downscaling leading to a preserved hyperexcitability increase in the likelihood of seizures.

As a practical consequence, one needs to realize the impossibility of a real assessment of MTLE patients without sleep studies. From a theoretical point of view, one has to keep in mind the importance of SWS in the development, activity, and prognosis of MTLE.

SOME THERAPEUTIC CONSIDERATIONS

Based on the assumed impact of interictal spiking during SWS on the insidiously developing memory deficit of our patients, one needs to look for new therapeutic tools. Our antiepileptic drugs do not inhibit interictal spiking, although concerning the new drugs and all kinds of IEDs, there were no systematic studies performed. Another new line of thinking could be to restore the loss of slow waves or to supplement slow waves to support sleep plastic functions (Bellesi et al., 2014). Some trials tried boosting SWS and increasing cognitive functioning in that way, but we are at just the beginning of a long work in this field.

DISTURBANCES IN THE HIPPOCAMPAL DECLARATIVE MEMORY SYSTEM IN MEDIAL TEMPORAL LOBE EPILEPSY

The most prominent memory disturbance seen in MTLE is the side-specific memory deficit. In MTLE affecting the dominant side, there are deficits in declarative verbal memory consolidation as well as in the newly learned material's recall. In MTLE of the nondominant hemisphere, there is a less clear visuospatial memory deficit, possibly due to either the insufficient visuospatial test battery or the unknown details of the bilateral organization of memory functions. The presence of an atypical hemispheric speech dominance makes the lateralization of memory loss more complex (Helmstaedter et al., 1999). The extent of memory loss correlates with several factors, e.g., hippocampal damage (Baxendale et al., 1998; Sawrie et al., 2001), bilateral involvement, the severity of the epilepsy, the number of generalized tonic–clonic seizures, the patient's age when the hippocampal lesion developed, and the amount of mental reserve capacity.

Side-specific memory disturbance mainly relates to early hippocampal injury. The structural changes cause an epileptic transformation rendering the hippocampus—or at least certain parts of it (Sano and Malamud, 1953; Margerison and Corsellis, 1966)—a discharging fireball, continually ejecting spikes and seizures, impairing the memory functions during periods of increased discharge rate, mainly during SWS.

Traditional textbooks have not paid attention to the important correlation of memory disturbances with the activation of IEDs during NREM sleep occurring every night. The hidden nature of the increased sleep-related IED rate and the cognitive decline in MTLE may be explained by the relatively late development of standard neuropsychological memory testing and—even more importantly—by the use of neuropsychological batteries almost exclusively in presurgical investigations. Another explanation might be the hidden place of the structures harboring the pathological impulse traffic responsible for memory disturbances. Owing to this covered localization, the activity of these structures was not detectable by scalp electrodes; it has become known only by intracranial and intracerebral electrodes applied during presurgical evaluations.

One needs to pay more attention to the interpretation of MTLE symptoms, focusing on their relationship to the memory system. It is obvious that the déjà vu and jamais vu auras are episodic memory symptoms, and Jackson's dreamy state may be consistent with a pathological memory state as well. One may wonder, are the orovisceral, emotional, and autonomic automatisms also linked to the memory system? It is also likely that the peculiar "impairment of consciousness" of complex partial seizures is more related to the memory system than we have expected. The impairment of contact with the environment during complex partial seizures with no loss of body tone and preserved orientation might have originated from the interference with memory recall, disabling the recognition of the environment and interrupting even self-identity without a global loss of "consciousness."

Several additional factors, like a speech disturbance or hallucinations strongly distracting the attention of the patient, may cause a loss of contact with the environment; it is hard to identify the actual responsible cause.

MTLE patients are usually unable to gain back their orientation immediately after seizure termination; their reorientation may be slow and gradual. The amnestic features dominate this reorientation period also and a complete amnesia for the seizure event is frequent as well. The degrees of the disturbance are variable and the roles of the contralateral temporal structures, the thalamus (Lee et al., 2002), and the broader frontoparietal fields (Blumenfeld et al., 2004) are unclear.

During the recovery period several postictal automatisms can be seen, e.g., nose wiping, face stroke, genital manipulations (especially in males), setting of clothing, etc. These automatic motor actions and behaviors are "lateralization" (side-defining) signs for homolateral seizure activity (the motor activity and the seizure are on the same side). This lateralization feature is probably because reorientation-related motor activity is easier to initiate on the homolateral side of the seizure than contralaterally, where a postictal paresis, subtle disturbances of motility, or neglect may compromise limb movements. If the "speaking" (generally left) hemisphere produces the seizure, the patient may remain unable to speak for a long period.

Hughlings Jackson, the first master of epileptology, recognized the "psychic aura" or "intellectual aura," also called the "dreamy state," in MTLE. It is characterized by a peculiar double existence is which a past experience emerges spontaneously, e.g., in the form of a hallucination (some scenes that had happened during childhood may be vividly experienced by the adult patient as a parallel reality, resulting in "double consciousness"). Jackson localized the dreamy state with anatomical precision to the uncus hippocampi by working up the temporal lobe of his famous patient Z, treated by him for several years before the patient died: Jackson found a small cystic lesion at the uncus hippocampi (Jackson, 1958). Penfield, in Montreal, who introduced epilepsy surgery as a standard treatment option, could elicit these kinds of delusions by stimulating the exposed cortex of the epileptic patients with an electrical current (Penfield and Jasper, 1958) in the operating theater. Later Bancaud et al., performing stereotactic surgery in epilepsy, showed the involvement of a more extended neuronal network including the amygdala, hippocampus, and temporal cortex, far exceeding the uncal hippocampal area identified by Jackson or elicited by the circumscribed stimulation performed by Penfield (Bancaud et al., 1994).

Those surgical trials in the early 1950s, aiming to treat bitemporal MTLE with bilateral temporal lobe resections, concluded in tragic memory impairments, providing lessons to the whole epileptology community about the essential role of the temporal structures, especially the hippocampus, in memory functions (Scoville and Milner, 1957).

Fell et al. (2001) were the first to show transitory gamma synchronization in the rhinal cortex and the hippocampus during successful learning of declarative memory tasks, by using hippocampal deep electrodes for presurgical investigations in the Bonn Epilepsy Center. Increasing evidence has since shown that in addition to local mediotemporal structures (connected to memory functions), a gamma synchronization develops also in the cortex during cognitive tasks (Llinas and Ribary, 1993; Cantero et al., 2004). Cantero et al. found that the gamma coherence is higher during wakefulness than in SWS or in rapid eye movement (REM) sleep. They assumed that the decrease in gamma coupling during SWS might underlie the decrease in cognitive functions, resulting in the difficulty in remembering our dreams (Fell et al., 2003). This assumption is supported by the finding that the loss of dreams is proportional to the time spent in NREM sleep between the time of dreaming and awakening.

COMORBIDITY OF MEDIAL TEMPORAL LOBE EPILEPSY AND DEPRESSION

Based on to increasing congruent evidence, depression is the most frequent comorbid psychiatric condition in MTLE (Altshuler et al., 1999; Kanner and Palac, 2002; Kanner, 2003; Błaszczyk and Czuczwar, 2016; Mula, 2017). The occurrence of depression seems higher in temporal lobe epilepsy (TLE) compared to other epilepsies (Piazzini et al., 2001), and it is especially frequent in left-sided TLE (Robertson, 1997). The disturbances in memory and mood associate with and mutually aggravate one another in MTLE (Helmstaedter et al., 2002). From another approach dysfunctions of hippocampal and amygdalar structures have been shown in patients with depression and specifically in major depression (Briellmann et al., 2007). Furthermore, several observations have found serious hippocampal and memory dysfunctions in depressive patients (Baxendale et al., 2005). Last, to close the ring, the link between MTLE and memory disturbances is also well known (Buzsáki, 2015). Therefore, here we face a bidirectional triangling situation between MTLE, depression, and memory dysfunctions, with a whirlpool-like strengthening of the malfunctions in these three conditions. Some data show that depression may forecast an epileptic disorder in the future, and low episodic memory performance is a premorbid marker of depression (Airaksinen et al., 2007).

Kanner (2004) proposed considering major depression and bipolar disorders as neurology conditions with psychiatric symptoms.

We also have to change our approach toward the most frequent psychiatric complication of MTLE, which seems to be linked essentially with memory functions, in which NREM sleep has an important causative role (Afridi et al., 2001; Antikainen et al., 2001; Marazziti et al., 2010, Darcet et al., 2011; Barnes et al., 2017).

THE CLASSICAL ELECTROCLINICAL SYMPTOMS OF MEDIAL TEMPORAL LOBE EPILEPSY

MTLE is the prototype of those epilepsies in which an early initial precipitator injury (IPI) is the first "hit," followed several years later by epilepsy as a second hit. The IPI is an early damage of the hippocampus in 60%–80% of cases. Typically, the hippocampal head is damaged by a complicated febrile convulsion evolving before the age of 5. The subsequent synaptic transformation, the neuronal loss, and the concomitant gliotic transformations result in a highly epileptogenic structure (Fig. 5.4) called "hippocampal sclerosis" (HS). Because the first insult does not cause

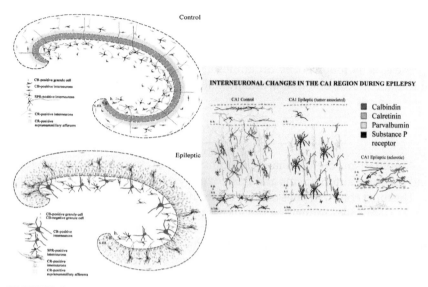

FIGURE 5.4 Drawing of the synaptic transformation of the sclerotic hippocampus in medial temporal lobe epilepsy patients, based on resected human surgery samples (work of Z. Maglóczky). *CB*, calbindin; *CR*, calretinin; *SPR*, substance P receptor.

immediate clinical consequences, it remains hidden; but neuroimaging may easily identify HS, the typical substrate of the epilepsy, producing seizures later. In addition to febrile convulsions, other causes (benign tumors, focal cortical dysplasia, cavernomas, autoimmune conditions, etc.) may underlie the epileptogenic transformation of the hippocampus. In addition to the hippocampus, the amygdala and the temporopolar cortical structures are also often involved. These coaffections of the temporal structures may accompany the hippocampal transformation or develop later as parts of a progressive process.

SEIZURES ARE OFTEN PRELUDED BY AURAS

The typical aura in MTLE is an uprising gastric sensation, joined by fear in 67% (Henkel et al., 2002). Jamais vu/déjà vu experiences may occur in 20%–30%; auras with olfactory and taste sensations are more seldom (<5%). Patients may lose their aura if the seizure-onset zone escalates in the course of the disease.

The characteristic seizure type may have different semiology depending on the affected side: dominant or nondominant hemisphere. Seizures starting in and involving the dominant temporal lobe have very rich semiology. In most cases, a motionless stare (an arrest) is the first step after the aura: the contact of the patient and the environment is suspended. The arrest may be reactive or areactive, depending on the degree of responsiveness. It is followed by an amnesia for this short period; meanwhile automatic motor, emotional, and autonomic actions may take place.

AUTOMATISMS

Automatisms are peculiar symptoms of MTLE seizures. There are ictal and postictal automatisms and "reactive" versus "de novo" automatisms.

The most common ones are those automatisms related to the oroalimentary system, like munching, swallowing, and chewing. Gastrointestinal phenomena like eructation are less common. Another "package" of automatisms involves variable autonomic phenomena like palpitations and changes in the heart rate or respiration, sweating, changes in color, goose bumps (erection of hairs on different body parts—piloerection), and shivering. Emotional phenomena make another special group, presenting with facial expressions and gestures like laughing and smiling or—most typically—fear. Nondominant-side MTLE seizures often manifest peculiar automatic speech expressing emotions, especially fear. The occurrence of emotional symptoms is understandable in view of the regulatory role of the temporal lobe and the associated limbic system in the ancient visceral, autonomic, and emotional functions.

Automatic movements, which may be very simple, repetitive, sometimes rhythmic ones like clapping, arm circling, or pats or complex activities like cleaning, ordering, or dressing, constitute another group. All automatisms present the fragments of one's everyday trained behaviors, "subroutines," appearing during the seizures unpurposefully, in an inappropriate way, place, and time.

The automatisms have remained the most enigmatic, unexplored semiological features of MTLE. The existence of "stored," automatized behavioral fragments helps us in everyday life to act "automatically," instantly with no preparatory time, when in need of a prompt action. These subroutines may appear in repetitive iterating forms, with no function or purpose during seizures. The physiological background of epileptic automatisms is elusive. Although state dissociation (see Chapter 3) is a good candidate for a mechanism, its applicability to temporal lobe automatisms is dubious. Whereas the automatisms of arousal parasomnias and nocturnal frontal lobe epilepsy occur in sleep, during a partial and localized arousal, MTLE automatisms present during wakefulness in fully conscious states, with no confusion or speech dysfunction either, particularly during seizures of the nondominant temporal lobe (Ebner et al., 1995).

Blumenfeld et al. (2004) set up their "network inhibiting hypothesis" for the interpretation of state dissociation, based on EEG and functional neuroimaging studies. Analyzing ictal and postictal features in MTLE, they found the hyperperfusion of the seizing temporal lobe occurring together with the hypoperfusion of the rest of the neocortex, associated with bilateral neocortical slow activity resembling sleep or coma. The regions of slow activity did not overlap with the discharging regions, excluding postictal exhaustion. Simple partial seizures have shown less neocortical slow activity and the degree of the disturbance of consciousness was proportional to neocortical slow activity. Stimulation of the output structure of the hippocampus augmented the neocortical slow activity, whereas intersecting the fornix resulted in its absence.

The difference in the disturbance of consciousness regarding dominant- versus nondominant-side temporal lobe seizures has not been tested in the context of postictal neocortical slow-wave activity during the exhaustion of the temporal lobe. The Blumenfeld group hypothesized that the ictal temporal lobe excitation inhibits the arousal system, resulting in sleep-like neocortical slow activity creating a base for epileptic automatisms.

MOTOR SYMPTOMS

"Positive motor symptoms" resulting from the spread of seizure to the suprasylvian region may associate with a later phase of seizures. Clonic or tonic motor activity of the contralateral face and upper limb (primary motor area) or the contralateral version of the head or the eyes (precentral adversive area and eye fields) may represent such positive motor symptoms. The most common ictal motor symptom is the dystonic posturing of the contralateral upper limb, possibly consistent with the involvement of the basal ganglia (Kotagal, 1999). Generalized tonic–clonic seizures are seldom (practically never occurring in children) and they are more frequent during night sleep than wakefulness (Pavlova et al., 2004; Bernasconi et al., 1998).

WHAT IS THE DIFFERENCE BETWEEN THE SYMPTOMS OF DOMINANT AND NONDOMINANT SIDE SEIZURES?

There are major differences in the seizure semiology of attacks generated by the dominant versus the nondominant hemisphere. Numerous video–EEG analyses have been performed since the beginning of the 21st century in epilepsy patients who have been successfully operated on subsequently. The seizures starting and remaining within the non-dominant hemisphere rarely cause a disturbance of consciousness or an inability to speak. There is preserved speech contact apart from cases with contralateral spread. Ictal speech manifestations occur more often in nondominant seizures, and emotional symptoms are also more typical in this group, e.g., fear or panic attack-like phenomena, ictal smile, and orgasmic aura (both rare) (Fakhoury et al., 1994; Marks and Laxer, 1998; Leutmezer et al., 1998; Rosenow et al., 2001; Janszky et al., 2004). The automatisms associated with preserved consciousness are features of nondominant hemisphere seizures as well (Ebner et al., 1995). Dominant-side seizures are often associated with or followed by dysphasia clearly related to the seizure spread to the neighboring speech areas.

The most important lateralization value is provided by tonic or clonic motor phenomena. Late unilateral clonus or tonic motor signs, including unilateral upper limb dystonic posturing, as well as an adversion (of the head or trunk) suggest a contralateral seizure activity (Kotagal, 1999), whereas unilateral motor automatisms are generated by seizures of the same (homolateral) temporal side. Their complex, correlated analysis as performed by Dupont et al. (1999), confirming prior observations on dystonic posturing and motor automatisms, may augment the lateralization value of motor phenomena. They found that dystonic posturing and automatisms are both present in 60% of temporal lobe seizures. There is an age-related change in seizure semiology as well. Lateralization signs are slenderer in childhood (Holthausen, 2003), and the nonspecific semiology may render the recognition of MTLE difficult in early childhood (Wyllie et al., 1993). Whereas auras, arrests, and automatisms are typical in seizures of puberty and adulthood, in the infantile TLE, the attacks frequently present with epileptic spasms, and generalized seizures are frequent possibly because of brain stem involvement (Chugani and Conti, 1996). In early childhood, motor (clonic and tonic) seizures are common (Jayakar and Duchowny, 1990; Brockhaus and Elger, 1995; Fogarasi et al., 2002). Reports of auras are infrequent in children, but seizures typically start with a sudden behavioral change, fear, and abrupt suspension of activity (Nordli et al., 1997).

INTERICTAL ELECTROENCEPHALOGRAPHIC SYMPTOMS

The diagnostic power of the EEG depends on the method and montage applied: conventional scalp electrodes, supplemented or not by an inferior temporal montage, sphenoidal or foramen ovale (FO) electrodes used or not, recording in sleep or wakefulness.

There is a local slowing in the seizure-initiating zone in more than 60% of patients, independent of the etiology (Koutroumanidis et al., 1999). Temporal intermittent delta activity is another important lateralization sign (Di Gennaro et al., 2003). Anterior temporal sharp waves and spikes are the most typical. Mapping studies have found different topographic configurations of the spikes' potential field comparing MTLE and lateral temporal epilepsy (Ebersole, 2000). Temporal interictal spikes are bilateral, but independent in time in 40% of patients (Williamson et al., 1993). Bilateral spiking is typical in patients with contralateral seizure spread (Hennessy et al., 2001). In FO electrodes, spikes and bilateral spikes appear much more often than in scalp electrodes, especially during sleep (Clemens et al., 2003) (Fig. 5.5).

EEG registration performed during sleep may importantly augment the EEG's diagnostic yield in MTLE: NREM sleep activates the temporal spikes. Additionally, it helps in defining the proportion of right- and left-sided spikes. REM sleep contrarily suppresses spikes. The facilitating effect of NREM sleep stages on spikes is different in FO and scalp electrodes. Although deep SWS (stages 3 and 4) exerts the most important activating effect in scalp electrodes, the highest activation in FO electrodes is seen during NREM phase 2 (Clemens et al., 2003). Owing to the maturing brain's specific features, broad (wide potential

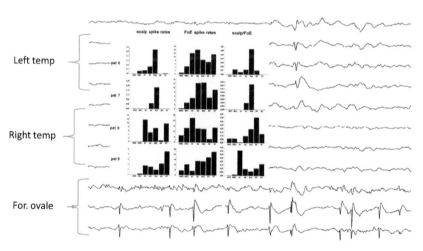

FIGURE 5.5 Foramen ovale (FO) and scalp spikes of medial temporal lobe epilepsy from four patients. When FO spikes coincide with scalp spikes, there is a time lag confirming the propagated nature of the scalp spikes. Insert: Histogram shows the scalp spike rate (left), the FO spike rate (middle), and the scalp/FO spike ratio (right). The number of spikes is higher during non–rapid eye movement (NREM) sleep in both the scalp and the FO spikes. The FO spikes highly outnumber the scalp spikes in NREM sleep.

field) hemispheric spikes, not temporal potentials, characterize child-hood TLE.

ICTAL ELECTROENCEPHALOGRAPHIC SIGNS

The seizure is usually heralded by the cessation of the interictal spikes, and immediately before the seizure start a desynchronization occurs. In line with the desynchronization, a characteristic local direct current (DC) shift best seen by corticography appears. Japanese authors 'have claimed for long,' the localizing value of the ictal DC shift (Ikeda et al., 1997). On the slope(s) of the DC shift, high-frequency oscillation (HFO) activity may appear. The coincidence of the shift and HFOs has high localizing value for the seizure-onset zone. Intracranial electrodes reflect more faithfully the seizure onset and the dynamism of seizure activity and allow picking up of gamma-range and HFO activity as well. The initial ictal EEG signs may sometimes be delta or slow theta bursts, and the 5- to 7-Hz theta or more rapid ictal repetitive activity develops later. This activity is frequent in the parasagittal line as well, appearing sometimes very initially in the sagittal electrodes, too. A contralateral spread to homologous temporal regions and to the parasagittal leads is common. The contralateral ictal rhythm frequently appears just in the parasagittal leads owing to a cingulate gyrus spread from the medio-temporal structures. The preictally suspended interictal spiking slowly rebuilds after the seizure (De Curtis and Avanzini, 2001). If contralat-eral seizure spread occurs, the postictal contralateral spiking intensifies (Gotman, 1991).

The electromorphologic presentation of mesiotemporal seizures is variable; there are several subtypes and their classification has been unresolved. Many researchers agree that seizures generated inside or outside the hippocampus are different. The multilevel signal-analytic methods helped by scalp and intracranial micro- and macroelectrodes applied in presurgical evaluation may provide new data and approaches (Wieser, 2004; Weiss et al., 2016). Seizure spread is an important factor in the genesis of semiology features. Based on deep electrode studies, the insular or laterotemporal structures involved in seizure spread generate some MTLE symptoms. The spread of seizures is slow in MTLE com-pared to the rest of the brain regions. The ways of contralateral spread are unclear. Seizures may spread to the contralateral mesial structures without the involvement of the ipsilateral temporal and frontoorbital cortex (Spencer et al., 1992; Adam et al., 2004). Possibly, the posterior hippocampal commissure conveys the seizures to the contralateral tem-poromedial structures (Gloor et al., 1993) (see later in this chapter in more details).

BILATERAL PHENOMENA IN MEDIAL TEMPORAL LOBE EPILEPSY

The research on MTLE over the years has supplied more and more data on the bilateral nature of changes, as suspected in early studies (Sano and Malamud, 1953; Margerison and Corsellis, 1966). Autopsy materials, MRI and functional MRI (fMRI) findings (Berkovic et al., 1991; Jack, 1994; Quigg et al., 1997), and later more sophisticated methods, including MR spectroscopy, have supported different degrees of bilateral structural involvement in MTLE (Seidenberg et al., 2005; Mackay et al., 2000; Eberhardt et al., 2000; Chernov et al., 2009). Fluorodeoxyglucose–positron emission tomography studies have shown bilateral hypometabolism in 20%–50% of patients (Joo et al., 2004). Bilateral spiking is trivial in MTLE, and the longer the recording is, the bigger the chance to detect them is. Different signs of Klüver–Bucy syndrome such as aggressivity and hyperorality have been described in MTLE seizures in case reports, suggesting a bilateral amygdalar dysfunction (Janszky et al., 2005).

Although the difference between uni- and bilateral MTLE seems straightforward, there is no clear-cut definition. Unilateral seizures, starting always on the same side, are widely considered "unilateral MTLE"; however, this concept does not take interictal electrographic symptoms, neuroimaging findings, neuropsychological results, etc., into account. The number of permissible contralateral seizures allowed in "unilateral epilepsy" is not defined either: where is the cutting point for calling it bilateral MTLE? The results of invasive studies have taught us that a scalp recording is often insufficient in localizing the onset of seizures. It is another lesson of invasive studies that there is an important discharge traffic between the two mediotemporal regions both ictally and interictally. These hidden aspects beyond the overt clinical seizure laterality point to the possibility that more contributing factors participate in determining the actual laterality constellation.

Connectivity studies have supported the importance of intertemporal interactions, too (Pittau et al., 2012; Bettus et al., 2009). Studies with shorter time span have revealed a low traffic between the homolateral hippocampus and the amygdala, even lower than between the two hippocampi, between the hippocampi and the mesolimbic dopaminergic system, and in the default mode network. Morgan et al. (2011) investigated the mutual interactions of the two hippocampi with high-resolution fMRI, using Granger causality. They have shown that the interhemispheric hippocampal connectivity and the Granger causality change time-dependently in MTLE. The connectivity diminishes first, and then it grows, linearly correlating with the yearly progression of the epilepsy process. Based on Granger causality data, the long-term increase in interhemispheric hippocampal connectivity is due to the effects of the contralateral hippocampus exerted on the ipsilateral one.

HOW DO BILATERAL PHENOMENA FIT INTO THE PATHOMECHANISM OF MEDIAL TEMPORAL LOBE EPILEPSY?

One explanation for the bilateral phenomena may be that the epileptogenic lesion had affected both temporal lobes. This assumption may be justified in postencephalitic or posttraumatic epilepsy; however, it is not generally valid: there are many clearly unilateral epileptogenic lesions presenting with bilateral functional changes, e.g., MTLE caused by temporal tumors.

Morrel demonstrated the mirror spike focus and worked out his theory about secondary temporal epileptogenesis on an MTLE patient series (Morrell, 1985). Animal models support the existence of the secondary temporal epileptogenesis; however, its validity in human TLE is not that clear, leastwise regarding seizure genesis. Bilateral spiking is common in MTLE, but it cannot unequivocally be linked with the progression of the disease, even if the presence of bilateral spike activity compromises surgical outcome (Hennessy et al., 2001), and also the postoperative persistence of contralateral spiking is related to poor surgical outcome (Halász et al., 2007). At the same time, bilateral independent spiking gets along well with unilateral seizure onset.

It seems exceptionally hard to demonstrate that a prior contralateral epileptic activity induces a unilateral seizure onset. To prove this, among other things, a follow-up video–EEG monitoring series would be necessary, but rarely achieved (Lüders, 2001). This seizure-generating process occurs very rarely and may need several years in humans (Halász et al., 2007). This rarity of contralateral seizure induction seems to parallel the waste of kindling across the phylogeny (Tsuru, 1981).

The significance of spikes and seizures in the mechanism of contralateral epileptogenesis is not clear, similar to the mutual interrelationship of spikes and seizures. Data suggest that the contralateral spread of seizures contributes to the evolution of contralateral interictal epileptiform phenomena (Janszky et al., 2001; Erőss et al., 2009). Seizures and IEDs are not synchronous; rather they alternate. Spiking generally ceases before, and intensifies after, seizures (Gotman, 1991), making postictal EEG recordings significant.

These data highlight the importance of seizure spread, even beyond its actual contribution to the symptoms of a given seizure. There is abundant experience on seizure propagation in MTLE; however, because of the hidden position of the medial structures, data that are more relevant may come from studies with FO or deep electrodes. The spiking registered on the scalp EEG is usually just a pale replica of the spike traffic detected with intracranial electrodes placed directly over the mesial structures (Fig. 5.5).

Bilateral mesiotemporal electrodes reveal very intense seizure propagation from one side to the other. The propagation depends on several factors, including the seizure intensity of the starter temporal lobe and the seizure propensity of the contralateral side, as well as the hippocampal pathology on any side (Spencer et al., 1992). The propagation time reflects the degree of coupling between the two sides, thus also having some forecasting value for the success of the planned surgery (Lieb and Babb, 1986; Spencer et al., 1992): fast propagation time would be an index for less success. Results reporting a decrease in interlobar connectivity—temporary interruption of the physiologic coupling between the two sides—at a unilateral seizure start have challenged this model (Faizo et al., 2014).

At the same time, FO electrode studies have shown that seizures starting in an FO electrode propagate the earliest to the contralateral one (Erőss et al., 2009). The route of traveling to the contralateral side has remained unknown because its investigation needs intracranial electrodes in humans.

There are contradictory tendencies in the ways and scale of interhemispheric cooperation across the phylogeny. The independence of the hemispheres appears to increase as marked by the suppression of the functioning of small association commissures, whereas the growth of the corpus callosum has resulted in a boom in interhemispheric traffic of information in primates (Jouandet and Gazzaniga, 1979; Wilson et al., 1991). There are several anatomic tracks of contralateral seizure spread: (1) the anterior commissure, (2) the frontobasal structures, (3) the posterior hippocampal commissure, (Fig. 5.6) and (4) the corpus callosum.

Spencer et al. (1992) performed the first deep electrode studies on spontaneous MTLE seizure propagation in humans. They found that of the 11 patients' 55 seizures starting in one of the temporal lobes, 4 evolved synchronously in the hippocampus and the neocortex, and 51(!) just in one

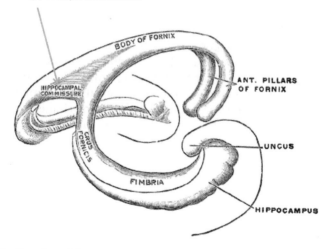

FIGURE 5.6   Drawing of the posterior hippocampal commissure between the posterior parts of the two fornices.

hippocampus. They detected three patterns of seizure spread: (1) from the hippocampus to the homolateral neocortex (32 seizures), (2) to the contralateral hippocampus first (13 seizures), and (3) concurrently to the contralateral hippocampus and the homolateral neocortex (10 seizures). The involvement of the contralateral neocortex occurred just through the contralateral hippocampus. These data suggest the activity of a human hippocampal commissure. We had similar experiences in FO investigations of 14 MTLE patients (unpublished data), recording 33 seizures starting in one of the FO electrodes. The seizure traveling time was the shortest between the two FO electrodes in 11 patients. The spread of seizures from the contralateral FO electrodes to the same-scalp leads was quicker than to the homolateral scalp leads in half of the patients. Direct spread to the contralateral scalp occurred in just three patients. Together with a contralateral FO spread, a simultaneous homolateral scalp spread also occurred in each case. The average propagation time was 6.1 s from an FO lead to the contralateral lead, 8.9 s from an FO electrode to one of the homolateral scalp electrodes, and 8.3 s from an FO electrode to the contralateral scalp. The studies of Gloor et al. (1993) on seizure spread and anatomic features highlight the involvement of the posterior hippocampal commissure in human MTLE. They showed that the anterior hippocampal commissure is rudimentary or absent in humans. A callosal route is unlikely with regard to the earliest seizure spread to the medial structures, typically seen long before the involvement of the neocortex. The role of the anterior commissure is more than improbable, too, given its lack shown by Gloor et al. (1993) and by others revealing the absence of an interamygdalar connection in primates (Demeter et al., 1985). However, more recent tensor imaging studies have referred to this traveling route again (Miro et al., 2015). The possibility of a frontobasal track has remained elusive because few studies have used simultaneous frontobasal and temporal electrodes (Lieb and Babb, 1986).

It seems unequivocal that the bilateral functional involvement in MTLE results in bitemporal functional changes. It is likely that the contralateral structures are not just passive objects of seizure spread; rather, they have an active role. It is clear that the two temporal lobes, especially the hippocampi and the amygdalae, work together also in normal conditions, sharing the limbic functions. The degree and mechanism of sharing or separating—bitemporal "splitting"—memory functions have remained elusive even though there are many related data at hand.

Based on the experience gained during the presurgical workup of MTLE patients there are abundant data on the bitemporal seizure dynamics:

(1) In the most common forms the seizures travel from one side to the contralateral side with variable latency (a matter of seconds). (2) Rarely, one side initiates the ictal state, continuing as a full-blown seizure on the other: the seizure-onset side is just a trigger, and the proper symptomatic seizure zone is the contralateral one (flip-flop mechanism). In such case the symptomatic contralateral side is not a passive recipient; rather, the epileptic excitability prevails in that side. Mintzer et al. (2004) presented several

cases in which the ictal changes on the scalp took place on the contralateral side while the detection with deep electrodes verified the seizure onset on the side of the severe hippocampal lesion. (3) Sometimes the epileptiform activity, including seizure onset, may manifest on the opposite side compared to the presumed epileptogenic lesion, e.g., tumor or trauma.

Further analysis of FO electrode recordings in our research group (Hajnal et al., 2014) has revealed peculiar dynamics after contralateral seizure propagation (Fig. 5.7). The bitemporal ictal electromorphological features differ from the usual seizure pattern, e.g., there is an increase in the amplitude and decrease in the frequency or continual tonic discharges occur, evolving to intermittent discharge clusters and seizure termination. If contralateral spreading has taken place, new seizure phases may start with unexpected frequency gain and amplitude loss. Sometimes the contralateral interictal discharges temporarily cease during seizures. All these changes are probable reflections of the mutual intertemporal lobe effects.

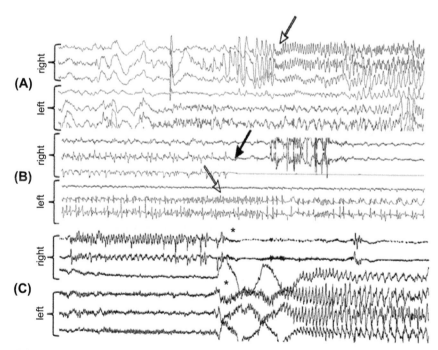

FIGURE 5.7 Intraictal changes involving both foramen ovale (FO) records. (A) *Empty arrow*, change in the frequency (higher) and amplitude (lower) in the left FO electrodes, consistent with a renewal of the ictal pattern ("autoinduction"). In other cases, in the contralateral propagated ictal activity the same changes may occur (not shown). (B) During left seizure activity (*empty arrow*) the right activity seems to be attenuated (*solid arrow*) like an inhibition. (C) Flip-flop pattern: after right-sided short serial discharges the right-sided seizure stops (ceases) and propagates (swaps) to the left side, where a more widespread and intensive ictal activity develops. The clinical seizure symptoms are congruent with the left-sided ictal activity.

By monitoring patients with bilateral independent temporal spiking and unilateral seizure onset, we found that the persistence of contralateral spikes was strongly associated with a poor surgical outcome (Halász et al., 2004).

LESSONS LEARNED FROM TEMPORAL LOBE SURGERY

At the beginning of the temporal lobe surgery epoch, most MTLE surgery was based on a noninvasive presurgical evaluation. The results seemed to be much better compared to pharmacotherapy (Engel, 1992, Wiebe et al., 2001); however, the success rate never exceeded 70%–80% of the operated patients, and the rate of permanent seizure freedom on no antiepileptic drugs was much lower (Téllez-Zenteno et al., 2005). The successful operations were variable-extension partial lobectomies, performed in patients with unilateral seizure onset on the scalp video–EEG (exhibiting congruent seizure semiology) with or without a neuroimaging lesion. Nonlesional patients had an unequivocally lower success rate. The methodology of presurgical evaluation, including sophisticated neuroimaging and EEG–neuroimaging fusion techniques, has become more accurate regarding seizures and interictal activity (including HFOs). The invasive approach helped to explore the relationships among the actors in MTLE, but more and contradictory data became known, rendering harder the selection of suitable surgical candidates.

Aghakhani et al. (2014), executing a wide publication search, systematically reviewed the literature on presurgically evaluated MTLE patients. They explored the congruency of MRI findings with seizure laterality on intracranial EEG and the seizure outcome of patients. One of the important results of this analysis was that 73% of patients supposed to have bilateral TLE based on scalp EEG findings proved to be unilateral after invasive EEG exploration, even after the exclusion of studies reporting a 90%–100% unilateral rate in TLE in their material. Fifty-eight percent of these patients had Engel I and 9% had Engel II outcome after unilateral surgery. Another conclusion based on outcome measures was that a bitemporal or ambiguous seizure onset is a weak predictor of bilateral TLE. Although unilateral patients had better outcome compared to bilateral patients, the degree of lateralization in those with bilateral seizure onset had a limited role in selecting the side of surgery. Overall, the seizure laterality seemed not to be the most relevant factor in the successful identification of seizure side in this big work.

Concerning uni- versus bilaterality, the interesting results of this thoughtful analysis suggest that bilateral seizures proved by invasive exploration and the proportion of seizure-onset side are not necessarily the leading aspects of surgical side selection.

We conclude that the side of seizure onset is just one of the aspects needed to be determined for surgery. For gaining quantitative markers of bilaterality, additional parameters and constellations, not directly connected to the seizures' side, need to be searched for. Such markers could be the interictal discharges with their HFO content, the spike-independent HFO data, the occurrences in the invasive electrodes during seizures, the laterality data of seizure termination, the dynamic features of ictal discharges, the lesional background, and the long-term data of progression.

We can build up a new approach on the bilateral existence of MTLE assuming a continuum of the two sides' roles. On one end of the continuum, we see the unilateral cases having the best surgical prognosis, and the independent bitemporal seizure-onset cases with surgical failures on the other. In the intermediate zone, the structures of both temporal lobes participate, presenting variable amounts of bilateral symptoms.

We propose to search for new indicators of bilateral participation. This new approach is beyond the surgical one, but is also beneficial for surgery. It needs to consider more factors, and make things more complex, but holds out to create a more coherent image of MTLE as a bilateral system epilepsy. It will shift our scope from the simple standard lobectomies to a more invasive approach and the use of stereotaxic techniques allowing better visualization of the spatial aspects of the epileptic networks.

THE COURSE OF MEDIAL TEMPORAL LOBE EPILEPSY

After infantile and early childhood febrile convulsions often observed in the MTLE population, the first epileptic seizures present in the second half of childhood, being seldom at that time. The first manifestation may be a generalized tonic–clonic seizure and it may remain the typical seizure type in the first disease phase. After this period, a relative decrease in the seizure frequency may follow, not surely related to the introduction of treatment. This "latent period" is not always there. After puberty, the frequency of partial seizures may increase and the attacks may be resistant to antiepileptic treatment. Secondary generalized seizures are rare, occurring more frequently just in severe cases. The seizure probability in adult MTLE is variable; antiepileptic treatment probably has an impact. Many researchers doubt if MTLE is a progressive condition, while others are convinced that it is (Hirsch et al., 1991; Didato et al., 2015). Several data support the progressive nature of MTLE (Pitkänen and Sutula, 2002; Sutula, 2004), e.g., the kindling model (Stafstrom and Sutula, 2005), the important synaptic reorganization shown in human surgical specimens (Fig. 5.3) (Maglóczky and Freund, 2005), the data on HFOs in experimental HS (Staba et al., 2007), and some MRI and MR spectroscopic studies. Bernasconi et al. (2002, 2005) and Lee et al. (1998) have shown a correlation between the duration of epilepsy and seizure-related temporocortical atrophy. The interictal neurophysiological features were shown to change progressively in only a few studies, but the presence of a progressive cognitive decline is unequivocal (Jokeit and Ebner, 1999, 2002; Nolan et al., 2004 Helmstaedter, 2002; Hermann, 2002, Oyegbile et al., 2004). At the same time, no correlation could be found between the duration of epilepsy and the degree of hippocampal/amygdalar atrophy on one hand and between seizure frequency, seizure duration, and seizure number versus MR spectroscopic changes (N-acetylaspartate to creatine ratio) on the other (Li et al., 2000; Burneo et al., 2004). Further, the proportion of bilateral epileptic manifestations has not increased with epilepsy duration either (Janszky et al., 2003).

The contradictory results of the long-term retrospective studies are related to inherent methodological difficulties. There are few prospective studies (Briellmann et al., 2002; Fuerst et al., 2003). These longitudinal volumetric studies revealed the progressive volume loss of the hippocampus over the years.

The antinomic data may be interpreted in such a way that after an initial pathogenetic event takes place, progressive changes occur in the mesiotemporal epileptogenic structures (especially in the hippocampus), and the very existence, dynamics, and factors of the further progression are unclear.

Medial Temporal Lobe Epilepsy Caused by Remote Extratemporal Lesions

In this form of TLE both seizures and interictal signs fully correspond to the known MTLE features; however, the underlying epileptogenic lesion is extratemporal. Based on the nature and localization of the lesion, there are several types.

Medial Temporal Lobe Epilepsy Caused by Peritrigonal Nodular Heterotopia

Peritrigonal nodular heterotopia is a human neuronal migration disorder in which many neurons destined for the cortex fail to migrate. This may be caused by the lack of a stop signal halting the neuronal development of the peritrigonal region, resulting in an overproduction of neurons or by a disturbance in migration itself. The epileptogenic change within the nodule probably relates to a GABAergic mechanism (Tassi et al., 2005). The heterotopia may have a diffuse unilateral subependymal position along the ventricles or be unilaterally dominant, mainly limited to the peritrigonal area (Battaglia et al., 1997). It is highly epileptogenic (more than 80% are associated with complex partial seizures), with interictal independent bitemporal spikes and a temporal ictal pattern on the EEG (Raymond et al., 1994). The familial and female preponderance suggests a genetic background in the first type, whereas the perinatal occurrence, bound to vessel-distribution areas, points to vascular risk factors in the second. The genetic transmission is X-linked (most males die prenatally) and the responsible mutation is in the filamin 1 (*FLN1*) gene; several additional genes may be involved (Sheen et al., 2001). Stereo–EEG studies have shown that the nodule and the corresponding dysgenetic cortex as well as the neighboring mesiotemporal structures may produce spikes. The cortex, the mesial structures, or the nodules can generate seizures; any combination may occur (Aghakhani et al., 2005).

Retrosplenial Tumor

We have seen in three patients that benign retrosplenial tumors may cause variable, including bitemporally located, spikes and temporal seizures. Surgical removal of the tumor has abolished both the seizures and the interictal EEG spikes (Halász et al., 2004).

Hypothalamus Hamartoma

The classical syndrome of hypothalamus hamartomas is the combination of precocious puberty, gelastic seizures, and psychopathological symptoms. Gelastic seizures are frequently associated with a temporal ictal pattern and uni- or bilateral interictal spikes. The ictal pattern is typically bilateral, but may also alternate between the two sides.

Sturge–Weber Syndrome (Encephalotrigeminal Angiomatosis)

The classical form of Sturge–Weber syndrome is an extensive posterior-dominant leptomeningeal angiomatosis in one hemisphere. The radiologic pattern of the calcified angioma seen even on the X-ray of the skull has a diagnostic value. Usually, it is highly epileptogenic and may lead to severe, pharmacoresistant childhood epileptic encephalopathy needing surgical intervention. Most patients can be diagnosed at first glance based on facial angioma (port wine stain; nevus flammeus) in the corresponding trigeminal innervation area. In addition to classical forms, computed tomography and MRI can also diagnose the milder cases. The nevus flammeus is not always present and the brain lesion may be smaller.

We had three cases in which a circumscribed posteriorly located Sturge–Weber-type angioma was associated with complex partial seizures, characteristic ictal and interictal MTLE EEG signs, and a homolateral HS.

These experiences suggest the existence of special locations and types of highly epileptogenic extratemporal lesions causing MTLE. How MTLE develops in such cases is unknown, but the involvement of the hippocampus is a common factor.

Apart from hypothalamic hamartoma also linked to the hippocampus, all lesions are in the posterior parietooccipital hemispheric regions, having abundant hippocampal connections. This is in line with the clinical observation that of childhood extratemporal epilepsies, the occipital ones may manifest MTLE semiologic features more often than frontal epilepsies do (Fogarasi et al., 2005).

MEDIAL TEMPORAL LOBE EPILEPSY AS A SYSTEM EPILEPSY

We have discussed in the previous chapters that MTLE ictal and interictal symptoms are determined by the physiologic memory and emotional system and, in an extended sense, MTLE is the epilepsy of the large limbic system.

The connectivity of the hippocampi and their association system is determinative in the formation of memory.

We have seen the important activation of the epileptic phenomena during SWS, expanding the spiking activity in time and space. This opens up and makes the whole memory system more permeable to epilepsy, impairing its sophisticated activity.

If this process affects the anterior amygdalar and cingulate parts of the limbic system, too, emotional symptoms may occur during seizures (as ictal fear in seizures of the nondominant amygdala) and interictally (e.g., easy buildup of fear conditioning). The frequent comorbidity of depression with MTLE also fits the concept of limbic system epilepsy.

As of this writing, interictal epileptic symptoms are mainly presented by records from superficial (scalp and cortical) leads. The more frequent application of deep electrode studies during preoperative investigations will provide extensive and three-dimensional data, highlighting the role of IEDs in emotional symptoms, anxiety, and visceral phenomena.

Connectivity investigations confirm the strong interconnections of the limbic system with the frontal and frontobasal regions known from classical anatomical studies (Reep, 1984). This is important in the interpretation of working memory disturbances experienced in TLE. It is likely that the fornix has an impact in the cooperation of the two sides (Jang and Kwon, 2014), and this cooperation might well be impaired by the MTLE-related abundance of pathological impulses conveyed by the fornix (Fig. 5.8).

The function of the insula was largely unknown, and it was the deep electrode studies that provided progress in this field (Isnard and Mauguiere, 2005). The studies on epileptic patients have highlighted that the insula is involved in the mechanism of pain and visceroception as well as those of several autonomic functions. It has pathological mutual interconnections with the mediotemporal structures, especially the amygdala.

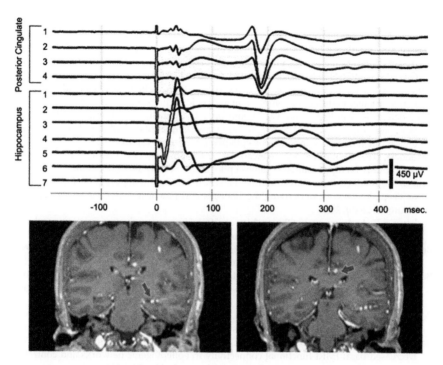

FIGURE 5.8 Medial temporal lobe epilepsy low-frequency stimulation of the fornix in mesiotemporal epilepsy (Koubeissi et al., 2013). The spike discharges elicited by fornix stimulation evoke responses in the hippocampus and the cingulate gyrus (the stimulation site is marked by a *dark arrow* on the MR images).

References

Adam, C., Hasboun, D., Clemenceau, S., Dupont, S., Baulac, M., Hazemann, P., 2004. Fast contralateral propagation of after-discharges induced by stimulation of medial temporal lobe. J. Clin. Neurophysiol. 21 (6), 399–403.

Afridi, M.I., Hina, M., Qureshi, I.S., Hussain, M., 2001. Cognitive disturbance comparison among drug-naïve depressed cases and healthy controls. Eur. Arch. Psychiatry Clin. Neurosci. 251 (1), 6–11.

Aghakhani, Y., Kinay, D., Gotman, J., et al., 2005. The role of periventricular nodular heterotopia in epileptogenesis. Brain 128 (Pt. 3), 641–651.

Aghakhani, Y., Liu, X., Jette, N., Wiebe, S., 2014. Epilepsy surgery in patients with bilateral temporal lobe seizures: a systematic review. Epilepsia 55 (12), 1892–1901.

Airaksinen, E., Wahlin, A., Forsell, Y., Larsson, M., 2007. Low episodic memory performance as a premorbid marker of depression: evidence from a 3-year follow-up. Acta Psychiatr. Scand. 115 (6), 458–465.

Altshuler, L., Rausch, R., Delrahim, S., Kay, J., Crandall, P., 1999 Fall. Temporal lobe epilepsy, temporal lobectomy, and major depression. J. Neuropsychiatry Clin. Neurosci. 11 (4), 436–443.

Antikainen, R., Hänninen, T., Honkalampi, K., Hintikka, J., Koivumaa-Honkanen, H., Tanskanen, A., Viinamäki, H., 2001. Mood improvement reduces memory complaints in depressed patients. Eur. Arch. Psychiatry Clin. Neurosci. 251 (1), 6–11.

Bancaud, J., Brunet-Bourgin, F., Chauvel, P., Halgren, E., 1994. Anatomical origin of déjà vu and vivid 'memories' in human temporal lobe epilepsy. Brain 117 (Pt. 1), 71–90.

Barnes, A.K., Smith, S.B., Datta, S., 2017 6. Beyond emotional and spatial processes: cognitive dysfunction in a depressive phenotype produced by long photoperiod exposure. PLoS One 12 (1), e0170032 Pharmaceuticals (Basel). 2016 17;9 (1).

Battaglia, G., Granata, T., Farina, L., D'Incerti, L., Franceschetti, S., Avanzini, G., 1997. Periventricular nodular heterotopia: epileptogenic findings. Epilepsia 38 (11), 1173–1182.

Baxendale, S.A., van Paesschen, W., Thompson, P.J., Connelly, A., Duncan, J.S., Harkness, W.F., Shorvon, S.D., 1998. The relationship between quantitative MRI and neuropsychological functioning in temporal lobe epilepsy. Epilepsia 39 (2), 158–166.

Baxendale, S.A., Thompson, P.J., Duncan, J.S., 2005. Epilepsy & depression: the effects of comorbidity on hippocampal volume–a pilot study. Seizure 14 (6), 435–438.

Bellesi, M., Riedner, B.A., Garcia-Molina, G.N., Cirelli, C., Tononi, G., 2014. Enhancement of sleep slow waves: underlying mechanisms and practical consequences. Front. Syst. Neurosci. 28 (8), 208.

Berkovic, S.F., Andermann, F., Olivier, A., et al., 1991. Hippocampal sclerosis in temporal lobe epilepsy demonstrated by magnetic resonance imaging. Ann. Neurol. 29 (2), 175–182.

Bernasconi, A., Andermann, F., Cendes, F., Dubeau, F., Andermann, E., Olivier, A., 1998. Nocturnal temporal lobe epilepsy. Neurology 50 (6), 1772–1777.

Bernasconi, A., Tasch, E., Cendes, F., Li, L.M., Arnold, D.L., 2002. Proton magnetic resonance spectroscopic imaging suggests progressive neuronal damage in human temporal lobe epilepsy. Prog. Brain Res. 135, 297–304.

Bernasconi, N., Natsume, J., Bernasconi, A., 2005 26. Progression in temporal lobe epilepsy: differential atrophy in mesial temporal structures. Neurology 65 (2), 223–228.

Bettus, G., Guedj, E., Joyeux, F., Confort-Gouny, S., Soulier, E., Laguitton, V., et al., 2009. Decreased basal fMRI functional connectivity in epileptogenic networks and contralateral compensatory mechanisms. Hum. Brain Mapp. 30 (5), 1580–1589.

Blumenfeld, H., McNally, K.A., Vanderhill, S.D., et al., 2004. Positive and negative network correlations in temporal lobe epilepsy. Cereb. Cortex 14 (8), 892–902.

Boly, M., Jones, B., Findlay, G., Plumley, E., Mensen, A., Hermann, B., Tononi, G., Maganti, R., 2017. Alterd sleep homeostasis correlates with cognitive impairment in patients with focal epilepsy. Brain 140 (4), 1026–1040.

Born, J., 2010. Slow-wave sleep and the consolidation of long-term memory. World J. Biol. Psychiatry 11 (Suppl. 1), 16–21.

Born, J., Rasch, B., Gais, S., 2006. Sleep to remember. Neuroscientist 12 (5), 410–424.

Bower, M.R., Stead, M., Bower, R.S., Kucewicz, M.T., Sulc, V., Cimbalnik, J., et al., 2015. Evidence for consolidation of neural assemblies after seizures in humans. J. Neurosci. 35, 999–1010.

Briellmann, R.S., Berkovic, S.F., Syngeniotis, A., King, M.A., Jackson, G.D., 2002. Seizure-associated hippocampal volume loss: a longitudinal magnetic resonance study of temporal lobe epilepsy. Ann. Neurol. 51, 641–644.

Briellmann, R.S., Hopwood, M.J., Jackson, G.D., 2007. Major depression in temporal lobe epilepsy with hippocampal sclerosis: clinical and imaging correlates. J. Neurol. Neurosurg. Psychiatry 78 (11), 1226–1230.

Brockhaus, A., Elger, C.E., 1995. Complex partial seizures of temporal lobe origin in children of different age groups. Epilepsia 36, 1173–1181.

Brown, T.H., Chapman, P.F., Kairiss, E.W., Keenan, C.L., 1998. Long-term synaptic potentiation. Science 242 (4879), 724–728.

Burneo, J.G., Knowlton, R.C., Faught, E., Martin, R., Sawrie, S., Kuzniecky, R.I., 2004. Chronic temporal lobe epilepsy: spatial extent and degree of metabolic dysfunction studied with magnetic resonance spectroscopy (MRS). Epilepsy Res. 62, 119–124.

Buzsáki, G., 1986. Hippocampal sharp waves: their origin and significance. Brain Res. 398 (2), 242–252.

Buzsáki, G., 1996. The hippocampo-neocortical dialogue. Cereb. Cortex 6 (2), 81–92.

Buzsáki, G., 1998. Memory consolidation during sleep: a neurophysiological perspective. J. Sleep Res. 7 (Suppl 1), 17–23.

Buzsáki, G., 2015. Hippocampal sharp wave-ripple: a cognitive biomarker for episodic memory and planning. Hippocampus 1073–1188.

Błaszczyk, B., Czuczwar, S.J., 2016. Epilepsy coexisting with depression. Pharmacol. Rep. 68 (5), 1084–1092.

Cantero, J.L., Atienza, M., Madsen, J.R., Stickgold, R., 2004. Gamma EEG dynamics in neocortex and hippocampus during human wakefulness and sleep. Neuroimage 22 (3), 1271–1280.

Cheng, S., Frank, L.M., 2008 24. New experiences enhance coordinated neural activity in the hippocampus. Neuron 57 (2), 303–313.

Chernov, M.F., Ochiai, T., Ono, Y., Muragaki, Y., Yamane, F., Taira, T., Maruyama, T., Tanaka, M., Iseki, H., Kubo, O., Okada, Y., Hori, T., Takakura, K., 2009 15. Role of proton magnetic resonance spectroscopy in preoperative evaluation of patients with mesial temporal lobe epilepsy. J. Neurol. Sci. 285 (1–2), 212–219.

Chrobak, J.J., Buzsáki, G., 1996. High-frequency oscillations in the output networks of the hippocampal-entorhinal axis of the freely behaving rat. J. Neurosci. 16 (9), 3056–3066.

Chrobak, J.J., Buzsáki, G., 1998. Operational dynamics in the hippocampal-entorhinal axis. Neurosci. Biobehav Rev. 22 (2), 303–310.

Chugani, H.T., Conti, J.R., 1996. Etiologic classification of infantile spasms in 140 cases: role of positron emission tomography. J. Child. Neurol. 11, 44–48.

Clemens, Z., Janszky, J., Szucs, A., Békésy, M., Clemens, B., et al., 2003. Interictal epileptic spiking during sleep and wakefulness in mesial temporal lobe epilepsy: a comparative study of scalp and foramen ovale electrodes. Epilepsia 44 (2), 186–192.

Clemens, Z., Mölle, M., Eross, L., Jakus, R., Rásonyi, G., Halász, P., Born, J., 2011. Fine-tuned coupling between human parahippocampal ripples and sleep spindles. Eur. J. Neurosci. 33 (3), 511–520.

Csicsvari, J., Hirase, H., Czurkó, A., Mamiya, A., Buzsáki, G., 1999. Oscillatory coupling of hippocampal pyramidal cells and interneurons in the behaving eat. J. Neurosci. 19 (1), 274–287.

Darcet, F., Gardier, A.M., Gaillard, R., David, D.J., Guilloux, J.P., 2011. Cognitive dysfunction in major depressive disorder. A translational review in animal models of the disease. J. Coll. Physicians Surg. Pak. 21 (6), 351–355.

De Curtis, M., Avanzini, G., 2001. Interictal spikes in focal epileptogenesis. Prog. Neurobiol. 63 (5), 541–567.

Demeter, S., Rosene, D.L., Van Hoesen, G.W., 1985. Interhemispheric pathways of the hippocampal formation, presubiculum, and entorhinal and posterior parahippocampal cortices in the rhesus monkey: the structure and organization of the hippocampal commissures. J. Comp. Neurol. 233 (1), 30–47.

Didato, G., Chiesa, V., Villani, F., et al., 2015. Bitemporal epilepsy: a specificanatomo-electroclinical phenotype in the temporal lobe epilepsy spectrum. Seizure 112–119.

Di Gennaro, G., Quarato, P.P., Onorati, P., Colazza, G.B., Mari, F., et al., 2003. Localizing significance of temporal intermittent rhythmic delta activity (TIRDA) in drug resistant focal epilepsy. Clin. Neurophysiol. 114 (1), 70–78.

Diekelmann, S., Born, J., 2010. The memory function of sleep. Nat. Rev. Neurosci. 11 (2), 114–126.

Dupont, S., Semah, F., Boon, P., et al., 1999. Association of ipsilateral motor automatisms and contralateral dystonic posturing: a clinical feature differentiating medial from neocortical temporal lobe epilepsy. Arch. Neurol. 56 (8), 927–932.

Eberhardt, K.E., Stefan, H., Buchfelder, M., Pauli, E., Hopp, P., et al., 2000. The significance of bilateral CSI changes for the postoperative outcome in temporal lobe epilepsy. J. Comput. Assist. Tomogr. 24 (6), 919–926.

Ebersole, J.S., 2000. Sublobar localization of temporal neocortical epileptogenic foci by source modelling. Adv. Neurol. 84, 353–363.

Ebner, A., Dinner, D.S., Noachtar, S., Luders, H., 1995. Automatisms with preserved responsiveness: a lateralizing sign in psychomotor seizures. Neurology 45 (1), 61–64.

Engel Jr., J., 1992. Update on surgical treatment of the epilepsies. In: Summary of the Second International Palm Desert Conference on the Surgical Treatment of the Epilepsies.

Erőss, L., Entz, L., Fabó, D., Jakus, R., Szűcs, A., Rásonyi, G., Kelemen, A., Barcs, G., Juhos, V., Balogh, A., Barsi, P., Clemens, Z., Halász, P., 2009. Interhemispheric propagation of seizures in mesial temporal lobe epilepsy. Ideggyógy Sz 62 (9–10), 319–325.

Faizo, N.L., Burianová, H., Gray, M., Hocking, J., Galloway, G., Reutens, D., 2014. Identification of pre-spike network in patients with mesial temporal lobe epilepsy. Front. Neurol. 5, 222.

Fakhoury, T., Abou-Khalil, B., Peguero, E., 1994. Differentiating clinical features of right and left temporal lobe seizures. Epilepsia 35 (5), 1038–1044.

Feld, G.B., Diekelmann, S., 2015. Sleep smart-optimizing sleep for declarative learning and memory. Front. Psychol. 6, 622.

Fell, J., Klaver, P., Lehnertz, K., Grunwald, T., Schaller, C., et al., 2001. Human memory formation is accompanied by rhinal-hippocampal coupling and decoupling. Nat. Neurosci. 4 (12), 1259–1264.

Fell, J., Staedtgen, M., Burr, W., Kockelmann, E., Helmstaedter, C., Fernández, G., et al., 2003. Rhinal-hippocampal EEG coherence is reduced during human sleep. Eur. J. Neurosci. 18 (6), 1711–1716.

Fogarasi, A., Jokeit, H., Faveret, E., Janszky, J., Tuxhorn, I., 2002. The effect of age on seizure semiology in childhood temporal lobe epilepsy. Epilepsia 43, 638–643.

Fogarasi, A., Tuxhorn, I., Hegyi, M., Janszky, J., 2005. Predictive clinical factors for the differential diagnosis of childhood extratemporal seizures. Epilepsia 46, 1280–1285.

Fogel, S.M., Smith, C.T., 2011. The function of the sleep spindle: a physiological index of intelligence and a mechanism for sleep-dependent memory consolidation. Neurosci. Biobehav Rev. 35 (5), 1154–1165.

Foster, D.J., Wilson, M.A., 2006 30. Reverse replay of behavioural sequences in hippocampal place cells during the awake state. Nature 440 (7084), 680–683.

Frauscher, B., von Ellenrieder, N., Ferrari-Marinho, T., Avoli, M., Dubeau, F., et al., 2015. Facilitation of epileptic activity during sleep is mediated by high amplitude slow waves. Brain 138 (Pt. 6), 1629–1641.

Fuerst, D., Shah, J., Shah, A., Watson, C., 2003. Hippocampal sclerosis is a progressive disorder: a longitudinal volumetric MRI study. Ann. Neurol. 53, 413–416.

Gais, S., Mölle, M., Helms, K., 2002. Born learning-dependent increases in sleep spindle density. J. Neurosci. 22 (15), 6830–6834.

Gelinas, J.N., Khodagholy, D., Thesen, T., Devinsky, O., Buzsáki, G., 2016. Interictal epileptiform discharges induce hippocampal-cortical coupling in temporal lobe epilepsy. Nat. Med. 22 (6), 641–648.

Girardeau, G., Benchenane, K., Wiener, S.I., Buzsáki, G., Zugaro, M.B., 2009. Selective suppression of hippocampal ripples impairs spatial memory. Nat. Neurosci. 12 (10), 1222–1223.

Gloor, P., Salanova, V., Olivier, A., Quesney, L.F., 1993. The human dorsal hippocampal commissure, an anatomically identifiable and functional pathway. Brain 116 (Pt. 5), 1249–1273.

Gotman, J., 1991. Relationships between interictal spiking and seizures: human and experimental evidence. Can. J. Neurol. Sci. 18 (4 Suppl.), 573–576.

Gulyás, A.I., Freund, T.T., 2015. Generation of physiological and pathological high frequency oscillations: the role of perisomatic inhibition in sharp-wave ripple and interictal spike generation. Curr. Opin. Neurobiol. 31, 26–32.

Hajnal, B., Szelényi, N., Halász, P., Erőss, L., Fabó, D., 2014. Bilateral signs and surgical outcome. In: A Foramen Ovale Study in Medial Temporal Lobe Epileptic Patientsl, Hungarian Neurosurgery Conference.

Halász, P., Janszky, J., Rásonyi, G.Y., et al., 2004. Postoperative interictal spikes during sleep contralateral to the operated side is associated with unfavourable surgical outcome in patients with preoperative bitemporal spikes. Seizure 13 (7), 460–466.

Halász, P., Janszky, J., Kelemen, A., Barsi, P., Rásonyi, G., 2007 30. Late contralateral epileptogenesis after incomplete surgery in temporal lobe epilepsy followed across 18 years. Ideggyogy Sz. 60 (5–6), 251–256.

Hasselmo, M.E., 2006. The role of acetylcholine in learning and memory. Curr. Opin. Neurobiol. 16 (6), 710–715.

Helmstaedter, C., 2002. Effects of chronic epilepsy on declarative memory systems. Prog. Brain Res. 135, 439–453.

Helmstaedter, C., Kurthen, M., Elger, C.E., 1999. Sex differences in material-specific cognitive functions related to language dominance: an intracarotid amobarbital study in left temporal lobe epilepsy. Laterality 4 (1), 51–63.

Henkel, A., Noachtar, S., Pfander, M., Luders, H.O., 2002. The localizing value of the abdominal aura and its evolution: a study in focal epilepsies. Neurology 58 (2), 271–276.

Hennessy, M.J., Elwes, R.D., Honavar, M., Rabe-Hesketh, S., Binnie, C.D., et al., 2001. Predictors of outcome and pathological considerations in the surgical treatment of intractable epilepsy associated with temporal lobe lesions. J. Neurol. Neurosurg. Psychiatry 70 (4), 450–458.

Hermann, B., 2002. Memory function related to hippocampal imaging findings. Epilepsy Curr. 2 (1), 8–9.

Hirsch, L.J., Spencer, S.S., Spencer, D.D., Williamson, P.D., Mattson, R.H., 1991. Temporal lobectomy in patients with bitemporal epilepsy defined by depth electroencephalography. Ann. Neurol 30, 347–356.

Holthausen, H., 2003. Characteristics of the presurgical evaluation in children. Epilepsia 44 (Suppl. 8), S5.

Ikeda, A., Yazawa, S., Kunieda, T., Araki, K., Aoki, T., Hattori, H., Taki, W., Shibasaki, H., 1997. Scalp-recorded, ictal focal DC shift in a patient with tonic seizure. Epilepsia 38 (12), 1350–1354.

Isnard, J., Mauguiere, F., 2005. The insula in partial epilepsy. Rev. Neurol. 161, 17–26.

Jack Jr., C.R., 1994. MRI-based hippocampal volume measurements in epilepsy. Epilepsia 35 (Suppl. 6), S21–S29.

Jackson, J.H., 1958. In: Taylor, J. (Ed.). Taylor, J. (Ed.), Selected Writings of John Hughlings Jackson, vols. 1 and 2. Staples Press, London, England.

Jang, S.H., Kwon, H.G., 2014. Perspectives on the neural connectivity of the fornix in the human brain. Neural Regen. Res. 9 (15), 1434–1436.

Janszky, J., Fogarasi, A., Jokeit, H., Schulz, R., Hoppe, M., et al., 2001. Spatiotemporal relationship between seizure activity and interictal spikes in temporal lobe epilepsy. Epilepsy Res. 47 (3), 179–188.

Janszky, J., Ebner, A., Szupera, Z., Schulz, R., Hollo, A., Szűcs, A., Clemens, B., 2004. Orgasmic aura-a report of seven cases. Seizure 13 (6), 441–444.

Janszky, J., Fogarasi, A., Magalova, V., Tuxhorn, I., Ebner, A., 2005. Hyperorality in epileptic seizures: periictal incomplete Klüver-Bucy syndrome. Epilepsia 46, 1235–1240.

Jayakar, P., Duchowny, M.S., 1990. Complex partial seizures of temporal lobe origin in early childhood. J. Epilepsy 3 (Suppl.), 41–45.

Ji, D., Wilson, M.A., 2007. Coordinated memory replay in the visual cortex and hippocampus during sleep. Nat. Neurosci. 10 (1), 100–107.

Jokeit, H., Ebner, A., 1999. Long term effects of refractory temporal lobe epilepsy on cognitive abilities: a cross sectional study. J. Neurol. Neurosurg. Psychiatry 67 (1), 44–50.

Jokeit, H., Ebner, A., 2002. Effects of chronic epilepsy on intellectual functions. Prog. Brain Res. 135, 455–463.

Joo, E.Y., Lee, E.K., Tae, W.S., Hong, S.B., 2004. Unitemporal vs bitemporal hypometabolism in mesial temporal lobe epilepsy. Arch. Neurol. 61 (7), 1074–1078.

Jouandet, M.L., Gazzaniga, M.S., 1979. Cortical field of origin of the anterior commissure of the rhesus monkey. Exp. Neurol. 66 (2), 381–397.

Kanner, A.M., 2003 1. Depression in epilepsy: prevalence, clinical semiology, pathogenic mechanisms, and treatment. Biol. Psychiatry 54 (3), 388–398.

Kanner, A.M., 2004. Is major depression a neurologic disorder with psychiatric symptoms? Epilepsy Behav. 5 (5), 636–644.

Kanner, A.M., Palac, S., 2002. Neuropsychiatric complications of epilepsy. Curr. Neurol. Neurosci. Rep. 2 (4), 365–372.

Kotagal, P., 1999. Significance of dystonic posturing with unilateral automatisms. Arch. Neurol. 56 (8), 912–913.

Koubeissi, M.Z., Kahriman, E., Syed, T.U., Miller, J., Durand, D.M., 2013. Low-frequency electrical stimulation of a fiber tract in temporal lobe epilepsy. Ann. Neurol. 74 (2), 223–231.

Koutroumanidis, M., Martin-Miguel, C., Hennessy, M.J., Binnie, C.D., Elwes, R.D., et al., 1999. Significance of interictal temporal lobe delta activity for localization of the primary epileptogenic region. Neurology 53 (8), 1892.

Lee, J.W., Andermann, F., Dubeau, F., et al., 1998. Morphometric analysis of the temporal lobe in temporal lobe epilepsy. Epilepsia 39 (7), 727–736.

Lee, K.H., Meador, K.J., Park, Y.D., et al., 2002. Pathophysiology of altered consciousness during seizures: subtraction SPECT study. Neurology 59, 841–846.

Leutmezer, F., Serles, W., Lehrner, J., Pataraia, E., Zeiler, K., et al., 1998. Postictal nose wiping: a lateralizing sign in temporal lobe complex partial seizures. Neurology 51 (4), 1175–1177.

Lewis, P.A., Durrant, S.J., 2011. Overlapping memory replay during sleep builds cognitive schemata. Trends Cogn. Sci. 15 (8), 343–351.

Li, L.M., Cendes, F., Antel, S.B., et al., 2000. Prognostic value of proton magnetic resonance spectroscopic imaging for surgical outcome in patients with intractable temporal lobe epilepsy and bilateral hippocampal atrophy. Ann. Neurol. 47 (2), 195–200.

Lieb, J.P., Babb, T.L., 1986. Interhemispheric propagation time of human hippocampal seizures: II. Relationship to pathology and cell density. Epilepsia 27 (3), 294–300.

Llinás, R., Ribary, U., 1993. Coherent 40-Hz oscillation characterizes dream state in humans. Proc. Natl. Acad Sci. USA 90 (5), 2078–2081.

Lüders, H.O., 2001. Clinical evidence for secondary epileptogenesis. Int. Rev. Neurobiol. 45, 469–480.

Mackay, C.E., Webb, J.A., Eldridge, P.R., Chadwick, D.W., Whitehouse, G.H., Roberts, N., 2000. Quantitative magnetic resonance imaging in consecutive patients evaluated for surgical treatment of temporal lobe epilepsy. Magn. Reson. Imaging 18 (10), 1187–1199.

Maglóczky, Z., Freund, T.F., 2005. Impaired and repaired inhibitory circuits in the epileptic human hippocampus. Trends Neurosci. 28 (6), 334–340.

Marazziti, D., Consoli, G., Picchetti, M., Carlini, M., Faravelli, L., 2010 10. Cognitive impairment in major depression. Eur. J. Pharmacol. 626 (1), 83–86.

Margerison, J.H., Corsellis, J.A., 1966. Epilepsy and the temporal lobes. A clinical, electro-encephalographic and neuropathological study of the brain in epilepsy, with particular reference to the temporal lobes. Brain 89 (3), 499–530.

Marks Jr., W.J., Laxer, K.D., 1998. Semiology of temporal lobe seizures: value in lateralizing the seizure focus. Epilepsia 39 (7), 721–726.

Mintzer, S., Cendes, F., Soss, J., Andermann, F., Engel Jr., J., Dubeau, F., et al., 2004. Unilateral hippocampal sclerosis with contralateral temporal scalp ictal onset. Epilepsia 45 (7), 792–802.

Mölle, M., Born, J., 2011. Slow oscillations orchestrating fast oscillations and memory consolidation. Prog. Brain Res. 193, 93–110.

Morgan, V.L., Rogers, B.P., Sonmezturk, H.H., Gore, J.C., Abou-Khalil, B., 2011. Cross hippocampal influence in mesial temporal lobe epilepsy measured with high temporal resolution functional magnetic resonance imaging. Epilepsia 52 (9), 1741–1749.

Morrell, F., 1985. Secondary epileptogenesis in man. Arch. Neurol. 42 (4), 318–335.

Mula, M., April 2017. Depression in epilepsy. Curr. Opin. Neurol. 30 (2), 180–186.

Nádasdy, Z., 2000. Spike sequences and their consequences. J. Physiol. Paris 94 (5–6), 505–524.

Nolan, M.A., Redoblado, M.A., Lah, S., et al., 2004. Memory function in childhood epilepsy syndromes. J. Paed. Child. Health 40 (1–2), 20–27.

Nordli Jr., D.R., Bazil, C.W., Scheuer, M.L., Pedley, T.A., 1997. Recognition and classification of seizures in infants. Epilepsia 38, 553–560.

Oyegbile, T.O., Dow, C., Jones, J., Bell, B., Rutecki, P., et al., 2004. The nature and course of neuropsychological morbidity in chronic temporal lobe epilepsy. Neurology 62 (10), 1736–1742.

O'Neill, J., Senior, T.J., Allen, K., Huxter, J.R., Csicsvari, J., 2008. Reactivation of experience-dependent cell assembly patterns in the hippocampus. Nat. Neurosci. 11, 209–215.

Pavlova, M.K., Shea, S.A., Bromfield, E.B., 2004. Day/night patterns of focal seizures. Epilepsy Behav. 5 (1), 44–49.

Payne, J.D., Kensinger, E.A., 2011. Sleep leads to changes in the emotional memory trace: evidence from FMRI. J. Cogn. Neurosci. 23 (6), 1285–1297.

Penfield, W., Jasper, H., 1958. Epilepsy and the functional anatomy of the human brain. Little bro Jackson JH. In: Taylor, J. (Ed.). Taylor, J. (Ed.), Selected Writings of John Hughlings Jackson, vols. 1 and 2. Staples Press, London, England.

Piazzini, A., Canevini, M.P., Maggiori, G., Canger, R., 2001. Depression and anxiety in patients with epilepsy. Epilepsy Behav. 2 (5), 481–489.

Pitkänen, A., Sutula, T.P., 2002. Is epilepsy a progressive disorder? Prospects for new therapeutic approaches in temporal-lobe epilepsy. Lancet Neurol. 1 (3), 173–181.

Pittau, F., Grova, C., Moeller, F., Dubeau, F., Gotman, J., 2012. Patterns of altered functional connectivity in mesial temporal lobe epilepsy. Epilepsia 53 (6), 1013–1023.

Quigg, M., Bertram, E.H., Jackson, T., Laws, E., 1997. Volumetric magnetic resonance imaging evidence of bilateral hippocampal atrophy in mesial temporal lobe epilepsy. Epilepsia 38 (5), 588–594.

Raymond, A.A., Fish, D.R., Stevens, J.M., Sisodiya, S.M., Alsanjari, N., Shorvon, S.D., 1994. Subependymal heterotopia: a distinct neuronal migration disorder associated with epilepsy. J. Neurol. Neurosurg. Psychiatry 57 (10), 1195–1202.

Reep, R., 1984. Relationship between prefrontal and limbic cortex: a comparative anatomical review. Brain Behav. Evol. 25, 5–80.

Robertson, M.M., 1997. Suicide, parasuicide, and epilepsy. In: Engel, J., Pedley, T.A. (Eds.), Epilepsy: A Comprehensive Textbook. Lippincott-Raven, Philadelphia, pp. 2141–2151.

Rosenow, F., Hamer, H.M., Knake, S., Katsarou, N., Fritsch, B., et al., 2001. Lateralizing and localizing signs and symptoms of epileptic seizures: significance and application in clinical practice. Nervenarzt 72 (10), 743–749.

Sano, K., Malamud, N., 1953. Clinical significance of sclerosis of the cornu ammonis: ictal psychic phenomena. AMA Arch. Neurol. Psychiatry 70 (1), 40–53.

Sawrie, S.M., Martin, R.C., Knowlton, R., Faught, E., Gilliam, F., Kuzniecky, R., 2001. Relationships among hippocampal volumetry, proton magnetic resonance spectroscopy, and verbal memory in temporal lobe epilepsy. Epilepsia 42 (11), 1403–1407.

Schabus, M., Gruber, G., Parapatics, S., Sauter, C., Klösch, G., et al., 2004 15. Sleep spindles and their significance for declarative memory consolidation. Sleep 27 (8), 1479–1485.

Schlingloff, D., Káli, S., Freund, T.F., Hájos, N., Gulyás, A.I., 2014. Mechanisms of sharp wave initiation and ripple generation. J. Neurosci. 34 (34), 11385–11398.

Scoville, W.B., Milner, B., 1957. Loss of recent memory after bilateral hippocampal lesions. J. Neurol. Neurosurg. Psychiatry 20 (1), 11–21.

Seidenberg, M., Kelly, K.G., Parrish, J., Geary, E., Dow, C., Rutecki, P., et al., 2005. Ipsilateral and contralateral MRI volumetric abnormalities in chronic unilateral temporal lobe epilepsy and their clinical correlates. Epilepsia 46 (3), 420–430.

Shatskikh, T.N., Raghavendra, M., Zhao, Q., Cui, Z., Holmes, G.L., 2006. Electrical induction of spikes in the hippocampus impairs recognition capacity and spatial memory in rats. Epilepsy Behav. 9 (4), 549–556.

Sheen, V.L., Dixon, P.H., Fox, J.W., et al., 2001. Mutations in the Xlinked filamin 1 gene cause periventricular nodular heterotopia in males as well as in females. Hum. Mol. Genet. 10 (17), 1775–1783.

Siapas, A.G., Wilson, M.A., 1998. Coordinated interactions between hippocampal ripples and cortical spindles during slow-wave sleep. Neuron 21 (5), 1123–1128.

Spencer, S.S., Marks, D., Katz, A., Kim, J., Spencer, D.D., 1992. Anatomic correlates of inter-hippocampal seizure propagation time. Epilepsia 33 (5), 862–873.

Staba, R.J., Frighetto, L., Behnke, E.J., Mathern, G.W., Fields, T., Bragin, A., Ogren, J., Fried, I., Wilson, C.L., Engel Jr., J., 2007. Increased fast ripple to ripple ratios correlate with reduced hippocampal volumes and neuron loss in temporal lobe epilepsy patients. Epilepsia 48 (11), 2130–2138.

Stafstrom, C.E., Sutula, T.P., 2005. Models of epilepsy in the developing and adult brain: implications for neuroprotection. Epilepsy Behav. 7 (Suppl. 3), S18–S24.

Staresina, B.P., Bergmann, T.O., Bonnefond, M., van der Meij, R., Jensen, O., et al., 2015. Hierarchical nesting of slow oscillations, spindles and ripples in the human hippocampus during sleep. Nat. Neurosci. 18 (11), 1679–1686.

Stickgold, R., Walker, M.P., 2013. Sleep-dependent memory triage: evolving generalization through selective processing. Nat. Neurosci. 16 (2), 139–145. https://www.ncbi.nlm.nih.gov/pubmed/?term=Stickgold+R%2C+Walker+MP+2013.

Sutula, T.P., 2004. Mechanisms of epilepsy progression: current theories and perspectives from neuroplasticity in adulthood and development. Epilepsy Res. 60 (2–3), 161–171.

Tassi, L., Colombo, N., Cossu, M., et al., 2005. Electroclinical, MRI and neuropathological study of 10 patients with nodular heterotopia, with surgical outcomes. Brain 128 (Pt. 2), 321–337.

Téllez-Zenteno, J.F., Dhar, R., Wiebe, S., 2005. Long-term seizure outcomes following epilepsy surgery: a systematic review and meta-analysis. Brain 128 (Pt. 5), 1188–1198.

Tsuru, N., 1981. Phylogenesis and kindling. Folia Psychiatr. Neurol. Jpn 35 (3), 245–252.

Weiss, S.A., Alvarado-Rojas, C., Bragin, A., Behnke, E., Fields, T., et al., 2016. Ictal onset patterns of local field potentials, high frequency oscillations, and unit activity in human mesial temporal lobe epilepsy. Epilepsia 57 (1), 111–121.

Wiebe, S., Blume, W.T., Girvin, J.P., Eliasziw, M., 2001. Effectiveness and efficiency of surgery for temporal lobe epilepsy study group. A randomized, controlled trial of surgery for temporal-lobe epilepsy. N. Engl. J. Med. 345 (5), 311–318.

Wieser, H.G., 2004. ILAE Commission on Neurosurgery of Epilepsy, ILAE Commission Report, Medial temporal lobe epilepsy with hippocampal sclerosis. Epilepsia 45 (6), 695–714.

Williamson, P.D., French, J.A., Thadani, V.M., et al., 1993. Characteristics of medial temporal lobe epilepsy: II. Interictal and ictal scalp electroencephalography, neuropsychological testing, neuroimaging, surgical results, and pathology. Ann. Neurol. 34 (6), 781–787.

Wilson, M.A., McNaughton, B.L., 1994. Reactivation of hippocampal ensemble memories during sleep. Science 65 (5172), 676–679.

Wilson, C.L., Isokawa, M., Babb, T.L., Crandall, P.H., Levesque, M.F., Engel Jr., J., 1991. Functional connections in the human temporal lobe. II. Evidence for a loss of functional linkage between contralateral limbic structures. Exp. Brain Res. 85 (1), 174–187.

Wyllie, E., Chee, M., Granström, M.L., et al., 1993. Temporal lobe epilepsy in early childhood. Epilepsia 4, 859–868.

Idiopathic Polyfocal Hyperexcitability Conditions (HIEC) of Childhood and Their Transition to Electrical Status Epilepticus in Sleep

Sleep, Epilepsies, and Cognitive Impairment
http://dx.doi.org/10.1016/B978-0-12-812579-3.00006-6

117

The group of idiopathic regional (polyfocal) hyperexcitability conditions (HIECs) contains the most prevalent, genetically determined, age-dependent, nonlesional (idiopathic) childhood epilepsies (epileptic hyperexcitability syndromes) classified into three groups with several common basic features: (1) idiopathic childhood benign focal epilepsy with centrotemporal spikes (rolandic epilepsy), (2) early-onset benign occipital seizure susceptibility (Panayiotopoulos syndrome), and (3) late-onset childhood benign occipital epilepsy (Gastaut syndrome).

These syndromes share a good pharmacologic treatability and a lack of residual deficits after the cessation of seizures. Although tracing out some focal features based on seizure semiology and inrerictal epileptiform discharges (IEDs) (most linked to the perisylvian cognitive network), the interictal signs, especially in the first two types, are polyfocal/polyregional with temporarily changing localization. Their genetic transmission and the underlying genetic change are unclear. The findings suggest mutations causing transient corticodevelopmental and increased excitability. In autism spectrum disorder and attention deficit hyperactivity syndrome patients with no clinical epilepsy, there are similar interictal spikes during non–rapid eye movement (NREM) sleep.

ROLANDIC EPILEPSY (BENIGN AGE-DEPENDENT CHILDHOOD EPILEPSY WITH CENTROTEMPORAL SPIKES)

About 15%–28% of epilepsy patients suffer this type of epilepsy. There is a male dominance (6:4).

Seizures mostly appearing in NREM sleep start at age 2–13 years, 4–11 years in 60%–80% of cases, and they cease at age 5–18 years. The electroencephalographic signs may persist after seizure cessation. The definition of the syndrome had originally excluded any pathoanatomic background; the mental development is normal; however, in some cases it may occur in children with brain damage as well.

About one-quarter of patients have one or more family members presenting with seizures; and in one-third of them there are centrotemporal spikes carried by first-degree relatives. In addition, twin studies have supported the genetic background of the syndrome as well, but the responsible gene or genes are unknown. Studies have highlighted the possible role of the *SRPXA, GRIN2A,* and *ELP4* genes (Lesca et al., 2012; Rudolf et al., 2009; Reutlinger et al., 2010; Dimassi et al., 2014). The genetic analysis is importantly hindered by the age-related nature of both seizures and EEG signs, making the EEG testing of the patient's parents unreliable. On the other hand, the characteristic IEDs are present in the families of only 1/10 of patients suffering clinical seizures.

The typical seizure type is a partial motor attack affecting the face, but also faciobrachial, versive, and hemiconvulsive attacks are seen. Generalized tonic–clonic seizures—presumably secondarily generalized ones—may develop in about half of cases. Some of the typical facial motor seizures are preceded by somatosensory symptoms such as tingling of one side of the tongue, the inner surface of the cheek, or the gingiva; salivation is common. These seizure symptoms put the seizure-onset zone at the lower part of the central gyri, at its turning region into the sylvian fissure. This localization coincides with the potential field of the typical interictal spikes. The seizures, apart from generalized tonic–clonic ones, are not associated with a loss of consciousness; postictal motor deficits occur in 10%–20% of cases. A typical symptom of the facial attacks in seizures of the dominant hemisphere is speech arrest. Most seizures develop before sleep or shortly after; strictly sleep-related attacks occur in two-thirds of patients. The attacks are generally short (2–3 min) and rare (not more than one or two per year). Generally, a long period of seizure freedom follows repeat seizures.

The syndrome's identifying feature is the typical interictal EEG pattern (Fig. 6.1). High-voltage sharp waves in the centrotemporal region are seen, frequently occurring in clusters or runs closed by a typical slow wave. The discharges may occur equally on both sides and make

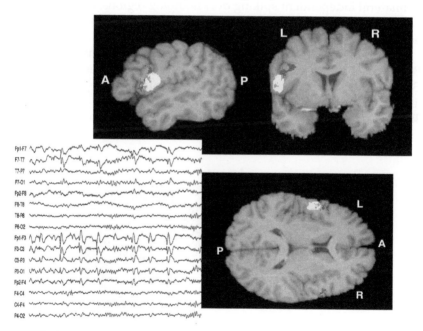

FIGURE 6.1 Benign centrotemporal epilepsy (BCTE) spikes on functional MRI. BCTE spikes are shown by spots of blood oxygen level–dependent activity (positive, yellow; negative, blue). *Inset:* The characteristic BCTE spike distribution on the scalp EEG. *A,* anterior; *L,* left; *P,* posterior; *R,* right. *Based on the work of Manganotti, P., Zanette, G., Beltramello, A., Puppini, G., Miniussi, C., Maravita, A., Santorum, E., Marzi, C.A., Fiaschi, A., Dalla Bernardina, B., 1998. Spike topography and functional magnetic resonance imaging (fMRI) in benign rolandic epilepsy with spikes evoked by tapping stimulation. Electroencephalogr. Clin. Neurophysiol. 107 (2), 88–92 with permission.*

up a bilateral independent pattern in half of cases. The centrotemporal potential field may shift to the frontal or parietal regions with no change in seizure semiology. The typical potential field is a frontotemporal dipole, localized perpendicular to the axis of the sylvian fissure (Fig. 6.2), whereas there are patients and age periods with parietal discharges. Mapping studies (Wong, 1991; Kanazawa et al., 2005; Yoshinaga et al., 2006) of rolandic epilepsy and Panayiotopoulos syndrome (PS) found that the dipole representing the interictal spikes appears around the big cortical sulci (the sylvian fissure, the parietooccipital sulcus, and the calcarine fissure) (in PS), i.e., the interictal hyperexcitability is localized. The third member of this group, Gastaut's occipital epilepsy, behaves somewhat differently. The unilateral EEG discharges are generally associated with the contralateral focal motor area; the hemisphere producing more discharges generates the seizures. In some cases, short generalized spike–waves may temporarily also occur during superficial sleep, and rarely in waking as well.

The topography of spikes is highly variable. In addition to the typical bilateral independent spiking over homolog regions, the distribution may be multifocal as well. Posterior variants may shift forward with increasing age.

Kobayashi et al. (2011) reported that benign centrotemporal epilepsy (BCTE) spikes are associated with high frequency oscillation (HFO) of 93.8–152.3 Hz (mean 126.2 ± 13.6 Hz). The occurrence of HFO was significantly higher near the seizures (Fig. 6.2). In atypical cases turning to electrical status epilepticus in sleep (ESES), proportional to the poor prognosis, HFO had higher voltage.

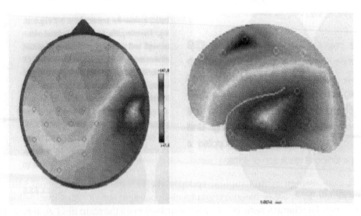

FIGURE 6.2 Amplitude-map of a typical centro-temporal spike discharge. The axis of the dipole is at the Sylvian fissure, the positive pole (green) over the frontal and the negative over the temporal lobe (red).

Slow-wave sleep (SWS) is the primary activating factor (promoter) of both seizures and interictal discharges. Clemens and Majoros (1987) found the strongest activation during deep SWS, especially on the descending slopes of the first sleep cycles. Nobili et al. (2001) and Beelke et al. (2000) have shown a more robust correlation of spikes and IEDs with spindling than with slow waves (Fig. 6.3). There was a similar correlation in Landau–Kleffner syndrome (Nobili et al., 2000). In accordance

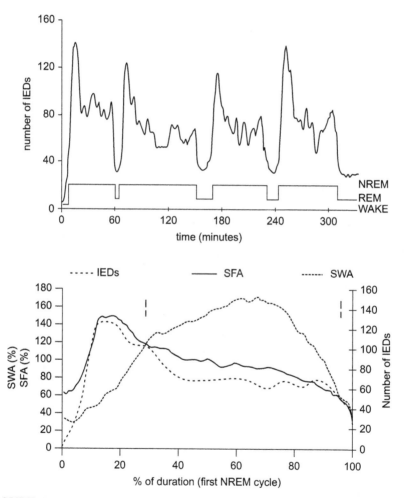

FIGURE 6.3   Top: Distribution of IEDs [benign centrotemporal epilepsy (BCTE) spikes] across sleep cycles. Bottom: Distribution of IEDs (*dashed line*), sigma band activity (*solid line*), and slow-wave activity (*gray dotted line*) in the percentage of the first cycle duration. It is clearly seen that the BCTE spikes associate with the sigma band—sleep spindles—and not with slow-wave activity. *NREM*, non–rapid eye movement; *REM*, rapid eye movement; *SFA*, sigma band activity; *SWA*, slow wave activity. *Based on Nobili's work with permission.*

with this finding the BCTE spikes of rolandic epilepsy, unlike the rest of the IEDs, are not activated by the A1 phase of the cyclic alternating pattern, confirming their non-slow-wave-related, but rather spindling-related, activation.

The occurrence of an atypical clinical outcome has been recognized: seizures that are more prevalent than in the benign majority of cases do not cease in puberty, and a cognitive deficit develops affecting learning, attention, and working memory. The EEG discharges are more frequent in such cases, completely dominating the cortical surface during sleep (see the section on ESES). Fejerman (2009) has named these cases "atypical rolandic epilepsy." The recognition of this atypical group has called attention to the mild cognitive symptoms affecting speech, learning, and working memory, occurring in typical benign cases as well (Verrotti et al., 2013; Besseling et al., 2013; Garzon, 2014; Vannest et al., 2015).

PANAYIOTOPOULOS SYNDROME

PS was described by Panayiotopoulos first in 1999; then he summarized and explicated further data and his concept on the syndrome in two additional papers (Panayiotopoulos, 1999, 2002). The syndromic spectrum and interpretation of PS have changed a great deal. A consensus report (Ferrie et al., 2006) published in 2006 characterized it as a "benign, age-related, focal type of epilepsy developing in early and mid-childhood. The seizures may be long with autonomic signs. The interictal EEG consists of multiple/changing localisation, most consequently occipital; morphologically BCTE-like discharges." Its prevalence in children under 6 years of age is 13% of all epilepsies. In three-quarters of cases, the seizures develop between 3 and 6 years and cease around 14–15 years. Two-thirds of them occur during sleep (Caraballo et al., 2007). Seizures may aggregate to status epilepticus. Most seizures manifest with autonomic signs. Vomiting attacks (nausea, retching, vomiting) make up 70%, but color changes, cyanosis, mydriasis, temperature changes, incontinence, salivation, vehement bowel movements, and syncope may associate or present independently. The autonomic signs may be associated with convulsions, hemiconvulsions, and atonia. Eye deviation as an initial symptom is not as frequent as was thought earlier. Seizures are not necessarily stereotyped; they last more than 30 min in half of cases.

The electromorphologic features are similar to BCTE spikes, occurring with variable localization and hemispheric participation. They are activated by SWS, but less so than in rolandic epilepsy. An occipital/occipitomedial potential field was most consistently found (Yoshinaga et al., 2006), related to the parietooccipital or the calcarine sulcus. There occur additional less consistent spiking regions as well. Despite the dominant occipital spiking field, the attacks do not originate here, first, because they present autonomic (vegetative) symptoms at seizure onset; second, because there are no ictal visual phenomena (in contrast to Gastaut's syndrome); and third, because the seizure-related tonic eye gaze is late if present at all within seizures. We have no proper functional anatomic interpretation of the semiology features.

The genetic background of the syndrome is unknown. Febrile convulsions historically occur in 17% of cases. PS may associate with rolandic epilepsy and Gastaut syndrome.

GASTAUT-TYPE BENIGN LATE-ONSET OCCIPITAL CHILDHOOD EPILEPSY

This smallest group, described by Gastaut (1982), constitutes about 2%–7% of childhood idiopathic focal epilepsies. Gastaut-type occipital childhood epilepsy (GOE) is also age dependent, occurring typically between 2 and 15 years of age with a nadir of onset around age 8 years. The gender ratio is equal. There is no brain-structural background. Thirty-seven percent of patients have a family involvement and migraine accompanies 16% of GOE cases.

The seizures present with visual hallucinations; ictal blindness may occur alone or associated with other ictal symptoms. The ictal hallucinatory images are typically small, colorful roundish patterns on the periphery of the visual field, tending to move to the opposite side. They grow and replicate in the course of the 1- to 3-min-lasting seizures and may be followed by eye deviation or ipsilateral head turning. Eye closure and blinking are rare. In cases of seizure spread to the temporal region, hallucinations that are more complex develop with unilateral motor symptoms seen also very sparsely. A migraine-like postictal headache with sickness is relatively common. The seizures occur usually in the daytime; they respond to "focal" antiepileptic drugs.

The interictal EEG features with occipital spikes and a slow closing wave, seen also in wakefulness, are mainly activated by SWS. Beelke et al. (2000) have shown a link of the spikes with sleep spindling similar to that seen in BCTE.

In clinical practice, the seizures need to be differentiated from migraine attacks. The visual hallucinations of GOE occur quickly, last a short time, and are colorful and circular; whereas migraine-related visual experiences develop slowly and gradually, last much longer, and are colorless and linear.

THE COMMON FEATURES OF HIEC

The three types of age-related hyperexcitability conditions have no brain-structural background. The functional anatomy features of the seizures are different in the three types, but the morphologies of the interictal epileptiform discharges are similar, and consistently polyregional with changing topography regarding BCTE and PS. In GOE, bilateral occipital discharges occur (but its special position seems to be less and less tenable).

Meletti et al. (2016) have published an EEG–functional MRI study mapping the network of the IEDs. They identified a bilateral occipitotemporal field involving both ventral and dorsal visual pathways and the fusiform cortices in 12 patients characterized by mixed clinical symptoms of PS and GOE, including those showing BCTE spiking as well. The positive blood oxygen level–dependent activity was proportional to the frequency of spikes. The primary visual cortex was spared. According to their interpretation, these results confirmed those earlier findings (Panayiotopoulos et al., 2008; Taylor et al., 2008; Sanchez Fernandez and Loddenkemper, 2012) suggesting that PS and GOE represent a neurobiology spectrum with overlapping electroclinical features and outcomes.

BCTE and PS may turn malignant, evolving to ESES, leading to an important cognitive deficit (see the next section on ESES). It is hard to assess the prevalence of ESES. It was noticed in just a few percent of idiopathic focal childhood epilepsies earlier, but is probably more than expected. Because of this condition's severe cognitive consequences, there is a pressing need to monitor atypical BCTE and PS children with sleep studies if there are any hints of an atypical course.

In BCTE and PS (GOE has not been investigated) the cooccurrence of HFO with spikes has been shown by Japanese researchers (Fig. 6.4). The quantity of HFO activity may forecast a disease progression to ESES (Kobayashi et al., 2010).

A malignant progression has great heuristic significance for highlighting the activating role of sleep in the pathology of epilepsy. Moreover, HIECs are good examples of purely genetic abnormalities underlying age-dependent transitory, MRI-negative developmental epilepsies. This pattern can be traced in Panayiotopoulos's term of childhood idiopathic "seizure susceptibility." The German Doose et al. (1996) had similar views earlier, considering HIECs a developmental disturbance. These conditions overlap with the group of well-known childhood

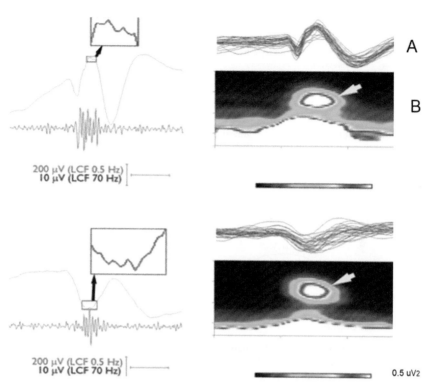

200 µV (LCF 0.5 Hz)
10 µV (LCF 70 Hz)

200 µV (LCF 0.5 Hz)
10 µV (LCF 70 Hz)

A

B

0.5 uV2

FIGURE 6.4   Ripples of ~70 Hz associated with spikes in a scalp-recorded EEG of continuous spike waves during sleep. (A) averaged EEG spikes, (B) high frequency spots (yellow arrows) above 120 Hz. LCF, low cut frequency. *After Kobayashi, K., Watanabe, Y., Inoue, T., Oka, M., Yoshinaga, H., Ohtsuka, Y., 2010. Scalp-recorded high-frequency oscillations in childhood sleep-induced electrical status epilepticus. Epilepsia 51 (10), 2190–2194 with permission.*

neurodevelopmental conditions like autism, tic–Tourette syndrome, and attention deficit hyperactivity syndrome, apparently occurring as the "cost" of the sophisticated human cortical development [the common EEG endophenotypes, e.g., benign centrotemporal spikes in NREM sleep (Fig. 6.5), are obvious markers of this overlap].

"Epileptic hyperexcitability" is a term used to characterize transient age-dependent focal, polyfocal, or polyregional interictal epileptic activity without epileptogenic lesions. It is difficult to adjust our localization-oriented concept with the existence of a variable, dynamically changing interictal activity of these conditions. Some cerebral gyri reaching simultaneously the same point of development or having more complicated developmental pathways may mark out the key points of polyfocal vulnerability where epileptic derailment easily occurs, possibly under dysgenic control.

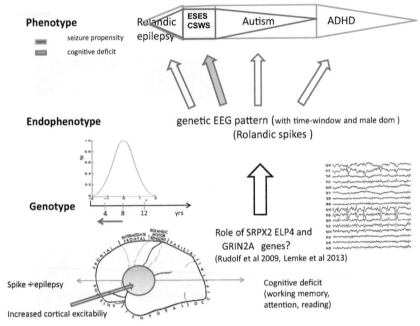

FIGURE 6.5   The EEG pattern of benign centrotemporal spikes as an endophenotypic feature shared by different epileptic and nonepileptic conditions. Top: Schematic representation of seizure propensity (red) and cognitive impairment (blue) in different phenotypes such as rolandic epilepsy, electrical status epilepticus in sleep (*ESES*)/continuous spike waves during sleep (*CSWS*), autism, and attention deficit hyperactivity syndrome (*ADHD*). The middle shows the age of occurrence curve of benign centrotemporal epilepsy (left) and the EEG pattern (right). Bottom: The territory of the *red circle* schematically represents the area of increased epileptic excitability and minimal cognitive deficits of the epilepsies like rolandic epilepsy. Right: The recognized gene-mutation types related to the EEG endophenotype.

THE TRANSFORMATION OF HIEC TO ESES (TASSINARI'S PENELOPE SYNDROME)

The Recognition of the Condition and Its Nosological Place

Childhood benign, nonlesional, focal/regional epilepsies are age dependent, gradually ceasing in puberty. However, since the 1990s several patients with a malignant disease course have been recognized: they developed severe cognitive deficits affecting just their speech or more global cognitive functions (Tassinari et al., 2000). It has turned out that their interictal activity had importantly augmented, flooding widely over the cortical convexities during all stages of NREM sleep, making a continuous electrical status epilepticus and causing severe cognitive harm. The treatment of this status epilepticus has been unresolved; the usual antiepileptic drugs are ineffective.

ESES was first recognized and described by Patry et al. (1971), reporting that it is nearly continuous during SWS, lasting for months or even years with no clinical seizures. The affected children suffer severe cognitive loss. Tassinari et al. (1977) considered it an "encephalopathy related to electric status epilepticus," supposing the causative role of the sleep-related status in the mental symptoms. The link with a deviant BCTE course was only later recognized (Dalla Bernardina et al., 1978, 1991; Saltik et al., 2005). In the meantime, acquired epileptic aphasia was also described and named Landau–Kleffner syndrome (LKS), honoring its first describers. It is also characterized by abundant epileptiform discharges during SWS. The affected children develop severe loss of speech perception after normal speech has evolved prior to the disease. Congruently, the spikes were focalized in the posterior temporal region of the dominant hemisphere (Kellermann, 1978), while no underlying lesion could be found.

It has become clear that LKS is a variant of ESES, in which sleep-related discharges focalize and interfere with speech functions.

We tried in 2005 to build up an extensive concept called "the perisylvian epileptic network" of benign focal childhood epilepsies transforming into the malignant encephalopathies LKS or ESES (Halász et al., 2005). In line with us, Fejerman (2009) have analyzed the features of the malignant disease process named by them as "atypical rolandic epilepsy." It seems more and more likely that BCTE, LKS, and ESES are consistent with different genetic variants of one disease, having different phenotypes in the form of focal childhood idiopathic epilepsies. The key factor in these epilepsies, regarding cognitive consequences, is the endophenotypic propensity to interictal activation during sleep (Fig. 6.6).

There is another aspect in the understanding of the ESES phenomenon, related to the condition's genetic/thalamic lesional background, calling for clarification. Since the 1990s, sporadic ESES cases associated with severe brain-structural lesions have been described. Polymicrogyria (mainly perisylvian) (Guerrini et al., 1998; Teixeira et al., 2007), hydrocephalus treated by a shunt in children (Veggiotti et al., 1999; Caraballo et al., 2008), and early thalamic lesions (Monteiro et al., 2001; Kelemen et al., 2006; Guzetta et al., 2005; Andrade-Machado, 2012; Quigg and Noachtar, 2012; Sánchez Fernández et al., 2012) have been reported on. We see now that more than half of ESES children suffer important brain-structural lesions; it is just the smaller half having a genetic background and developing from idiopathic focal childhood epilepsies. One may suppose that also in structural lesion cases still-unknown genetic predisposing factors contribute to the development of ESES. It is also possible that denervation sensitivity would be an important factor in the development of ESES in structural lesions, especially where early thalamic damage is present.

Early thalamic lesions are especially interesting as they suggest the impact of the thalamus and the thalamocortical system in the

AWAKE   SLEEP

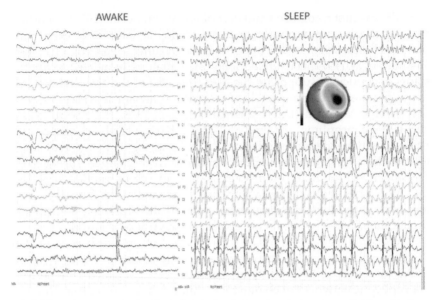

FIGURE 6.6   Atypical rolandic epilepsy turning to electrical status epilepticus in sleep (ESES) in non–rapid eye movement (NREM) sleep. Left: Waking state with sporadic centro-temporal single spikes. Right: The same patient during NREM sleep shaping ESES-type continuous discharges during NREM sleep. *Inset*: the localization of spikes shown by an average scalp voltage map during sleep, indicating a focal unihemispheric posterior centrotemporal negative field.

pathomechanism of ESES. There are contradicting epidemiology data: several papers suggest that in the majority of early thalamic lesion infants ESES may develop (e.g., Guzzetta et al., 2005), whereas of 32 ESES children at the Bethesda Children's Hospital Budapest, just four had thalamic lesions, and only one patient had it in isolation (Hegyi et al., 2016).

Sanchez Fernandez et al. (2012) supposed that the discharges of ESES considered as a spike–wave pattern "use" the sleep-related burst-firing mode of the thalamocortical system similar to absence epilepsy, based on the concept of Gloor (1968).

To discuss this, we need to clarify whether the discharges of ESES are really consistent with bilateral synchronous spike–waves.

The Features of Sleep-Related Discharges in ESES and the Mechanism of Their Activation During Slow-Wave Sleep

ESES is age dependent; it may start in early childhood and cease before puberty. Its most prominent feature is the abundant activation of epileptiform discharges, exclusively during SWS. The traditional definition of ESES had required the presence of pathologic discharges in 85%

of SWS. The present cutoff criterion is lower; 25%–85% of SWS covered by discharges is accepted for the diagnosis of ESES (Sanchez Fernandez et al., 2012).

The severity of the cognitive deficit in ESES appears to correlate with the duration of ESES, and the clinical reversibility depends on its disappearance. The topography of discharges (see later) determines the quality of cognitive deficit. In cases in which HIEC patients had sleep recordings before the progression to ESES, there were sleep IEDs similar to those in BCTE and PS, whereas during the ESES phase there were differences seen in the frequency, voltage, synchrony, and spread of the discharges.

Sleep activation has an uprising phase, a plateau, and a regressing phase. One may generally find the "leading hemisphere" producing the first discharges before the spread and carrying on in the end, for the longest time, during the regression phase (Fig. 6.7). The degree of the spread and contralateral propagation of regional discharges varies during the course of the disease, both within one and within the two hemispheres (Halász et al., 2014).

It has been shown by different methods that the propagation between homolog areas of the two hemispheres needs a transmission time, which underlies "secondary bilateral synchrony" (Tükel and Jasper, 1952). This is an EEG concept of the seemingly synchronous activation of the two hemispheres stating that there must be a secondary spread, a contralateral

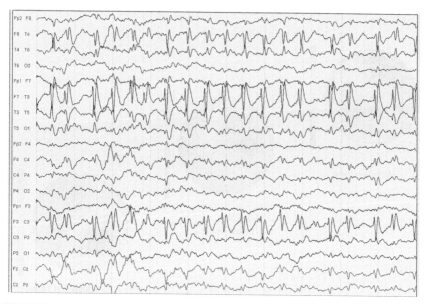

FIGURE 6.7 The electrical status epilepticus in sleep pattern is not always bilaterally symmetric: left-hemisphere temporocentral and independent right-hemisphere temporal regional distribution of the discharges are shown.

transmission behind the bilateral appearance of the discharges. It used to be attributed to a central (thalamic) pacemaker; this is not accepted anymore, and its anatomical bases are worn out, too.

In the ESES material of the Bethesda Hospital Budapest, we have found that the dipoles made by the discharges of ESES typically did not have a phase reversal over the central region of both hemispheres, unlike the well-known dipoles of spike–wave discharges of the bilateral spike–waves of absence epilepsy. Rather, the ESES discharges had a hemispheric dominance and a phase reversal over the axis of the sylvian fissure in both lesional and nonlesional cases (Halász et al., 2014) (Fig. 6.8).

We have seen in earlier sections that the IEDs of HIEC patients are importantly activated during SWS. Clemens and Majoros (1987) found the strongest activation of IEDs on the descending slopes of the first cycles of deep SWS. At the same time, in virtual contrast with this finding, unlike all the rest of the epilepsies, Terzano et al. (1991) found no temporal link between BCTE spikes and cyclic alternating pattern A1 phase, that is, with evoked slow waves. Rather, there were associations with sleep spindling as recognized also by other Italian researchers (Nobili et al., 1999; Beelke et al., 2000) (Fig. 6.3). Kellaway (2000) had earlier highlighted the relationship of sleep spindles and BCTE discharges as well.

The mechanism of the exceptional sleep activation of ESES is unknown. Possibly, the sleep activation seen also in idiopathic childhood focal epilepsies may trigger a kindling-like, epileptic "learning"

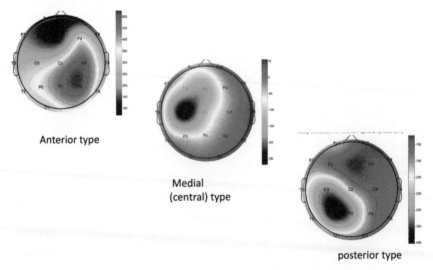

Anterior type

Medial
(central) type

posterior type

FIGURE 6.8 Characteristic focal potential-field variants of discharges situated along the sylvian fissure, constituting the majority of electrical status epilepticus in sleep patterns in our material (Halász et al., 2014) without or with cerebral lesion(s).

process in genetically susceptible patients. This may exaggerate the sleep activation: slowly, systematically, the kindling-like epileptic activation overwhelms widespread regions and patches, then insidiously spreads to both hemispheres involving the homolog regions. This pattern of activation might be underlain by a specific sleep-activation endophenotype. Sleep activation is a common feature in several other epilepsies. The variance of the amount of activation within the group of ESES patients is also congruent with the fact that ESES represents only an extreme variation of a more common phenomenon.

We can see more and more clearly that memory consolidation needs SWS as the pledge of earning (see later). This plastic function, memory consolidation, justifies the seemingly uneconomical presence and persistence of sleep across the phylogeny. Epileptic discharges interweaving SWS may interfere with its plastic functions, vividly depicted by Tassinari in the description of Penelope syndrome (Tassinari et al., 2009).[1]

Studies on the sleep of ESES patients indirectly suggest the lack of nighttime synaptic downscaling (Bölsterli et al., 2011; Cantalupo et al., 2011; Bigna et al., 2014). Another possible substrate of cognitive impairment in ESES patients is the possible epileptic transformation of the hippocampal gamma oscillations to a high-frequency oscillation, called (epileptic/pathologic) p-ripples (Buzsáki, 2015), linked to epileptic discharges (Kobayashi et al., 2010). P-ripples interfere with cognitive processing and memory consolidation (Buzsáki, 2015).

References

Andrade-Machado, R., 2012. Early thalamic lesions in patients with sleep-potentiated epileptiform activity. Neurology 79 (22), 2218.

Beelke, M., Nobili, L., Baglietto, M.G., De Carli, F., Robert, A., De Negri, E., Ferrillo, F., 2000. Relationship of sigma activity to sleep interictal epileptic discharges: a study in children affected by benign epilepsy with occipital paroxysms. Epilepsy Res. 40 (2–3), 179–186.

Besseling, R.M., Jansen, J.F., Overvliet, G.M., van der Kruijs, S.J., Vles, J.S., Ebus, S.C., Hofman, P.A., Ad, L., Aldenkamp, A.P., Backes, W.H., 2013. Reduced functional integration of the sensorimotor and language network in rolandic epilepsy. Neuroimage Clin. 2, 239–246.

Bigna, K., Bölsterli, H., Fattinger, S., Kurth, S., LeBourgeois, M.K., et al., 2014. Spike wave location and density disturb sleep slow waves in patients with CSWS (continuous spike waves during sleep). Epilepsia 55 (4), 584–591.

[1] In the legendary epos of Homer, *The Trojan War*, during the absence of Odysseus, Penelope, Odysseus's wife, told her suitors that she needed to weave her father-in-law's (Laertes) death shroud first, and she could choose from among the suitors only after. What she weaved during the day, she unraveled secretly during each night, delaying the time of decision. (*Analogy: what is built upon the neuronal networks during the day cannot be utilized because of the interference with nighttime spiking.*)

Bölsterli, B.K., Schmitt, B., Bast, T., Critelli, H., Heinzle, J., Jenni, O.G., Huber, R., 2011. Impaired slow wave sleep downscaling in encephalopathy with status epilepticus during sleep (ESES). Clin. Neurophysiol. 122 (9), 1779–1787.

Buzsáki, G., 2015. Hippocampal sharp wave-ripple: a cognitive biomarker for episodic memory and planning. Hippocampus 25 (10), 1073–1188.

Cantalupo, G., Rubboli, G., Tassinari, C.A., 2011. Night-time unravelling of the brain web: impaired synaptic downscaling in ESES-the Penelope syndrome. Clin. Neurophysiol. 122 (9), 1691–1692.

Caraballo, R., Cersósimo, R., Fejerman, N., 2007. Panayiotopoulos syndrome: a prospective study of 192 patients. Epilepsia 48 (6), 1054–1061.

Caraballo, R.H., Bongiorni, L., Cersósimo, R., Semprino, M., Espeche, A., Fejerman, N., 2008. Epileptic encephalopathy with continuous spikes and waves during sleep in children with shunted hydrocephalus: a study of nine cases. Epilepsia 49 (9), 1520–1527.

Clemens, B., Majoros, E., 1987. Sleep studies in benign epilepsy of childhood with rolandic spikes. II. Analysis of discharge frequency and its relation to sleep dynamics. Epilepsia 28 (1), 24–27.

Dalla Bernardina, B., Sgrò, V., Caraballo, R., Fontana, E., Colamaria, V., Zullini, E., Simone, M., Zanetti, R., 1991. Sleep and benign partial epilepsies of childhood: EEG and evoked potentials study. Epilepsy Res. Suppl. 2, 83–96.

Dalla Bernardina, B., Tassinari, C.A., Dravet, C., Bureau, M., Beghini, G., Roger, J., 1978. Benign focal epilepsy and "electrical status epilepticus" during sleep. Rev. Electroencephalogr. Neurophysiol. Clin. 8 (3), 350–353.

Dimassi, S., Labalme, A., Lesca, G., Rudolf, G., Bruneau, N., et al., 2014. A subset of genomic alterations detected in rolandic epilepsies contains candidate or known epilepsy genes including GRIN2A and PRRT2. Epilepsia 55 (2), 370–378.

Doose, H., Neubauer, B., Carlsson, G., 1996. Children with benign focal sharp waves in the EEG-developmental disorders and epilepsy. Neuropediatrics 27 (5), 227–241.

Fejerman, N., 2009. Atypical rolandic epilepsy. Epilepsia 50 (Suppl. 7), 9–12.

Ferrie, C., Caraballo, R., Covanis, A., Demirbilek, V., Dervent, A., Kivity, S., Koutroumanidis, M., Martinovic, Z., Oguni, H., Verrotti, A., Vigevano, F., Watanabe, K., Yalcin, D., Yoshinaga, H., 2006. Panayiotopoulos syndrome: a consensus view. Dev. Med. Child. Neurol. 48, 236–240.

Garzon, E., 2014. Is rolandic epilepsy really benign? Arq. Neuropsiquiatr. 72 (11), 821–823.

Gastaut, H., 1982. Benign spike-wave occipital epilepsy in children. Rev. Electroencephalogr. Neurophysiol. Clin. 12 (3), 179–201.

Gloor, P., 1968. Generalized cortico-reticular epilepsies, some considerations on the pathophysiology of generalized bilaterally synchronous spike and wave discharge. Epilepsia 9 (3), 249–263.

Guerrini, R., Genton, P., Bureau, M., Parmeggiani, A., Salas-Puig, X., Santucci, M., Bonanni, P., Ambrosetto, G., Dravet, C., 1998. Multilobar polymicrogyria, intractable drop attack seizures, and sleep-related electrical status epilepticus. Neurology 51 (2), 504–512.

Guzzetta, F., Battaglia, D., Veredice, C., Donvito, V., Pane, M., Lettori, D., Chiricozzi, F., Chieffo, D., Tartaglione, T., Dravet, C., 2005. Early thalamic injury associated with epilepsy and continuous spike-wave during slow sleep. Epilepsia 46 (6), 889–900.

Halász, P., Hegyi, M., Zs, S., Fogarasi, A., 2014. Encephalopathy with status electricus in slow wave sleep – a review with an emphasis on the regional (perisylvian) aspects. J. Epileptol. 22 (2), 71–87.

Halász, P., Kelemen, A., Clemens, B., Saracz, J., Rosdy, B., Rásonyi, G., Szűcs, A., 2005. The perisylvian epileptic network. A unifying concept. Ideggyogy. Szle. 58 (1–2), 21–31.

Hegyi, M., Siegler, Z., Fogarasi, A., Barsi, P., Halász, P., 2016. Long term follow-up of lesional and non-lesional patients with electrical status epilepticus in slow wave sleep. Ideggyógy. Szle. 69 (1–2).

Kanazawa, O., Tohyama, J., Akasaka, N., Kamimura, T., 2005. A magnetoencephalographic study of patients with Panayiotopoulos syndrome. Epilepsia 46 (7), 1106–1113.

Kelemen, A., Barsi, P., Gyorsok, Z., Sarac, J., Szűcs, A., Halász, P., 2006. Thalamic lesion and epilepsy with generalized seizures, ESES and spike-wave paroxysms-report of three cases. Seizure 15 (6), 454–458.

Kellaway, P., 2000. The electroencephalographic features of benign centrotemporal (rolandic) epilepsy of childhood. Epilepsia 41 (8), 1053–1056.

Kellermann, K., 1978. Recurrent aphasia with subclinical bioelectric status epilepticus during sleep. Eur. J. Pediatr. 128, 207–212.

Kobayashi, K., Watanabe, Y., Inoue, T., Oka, M., Yoshinaga, H., Ohtsuka, Y., 2010. Scalp-recorded high-frequency oscillations in childhood sleep-induced electrical status epilepticus. Epilepsia 51 (10), 2190–2194.

Lesca, G., Rudolf, G., Labalme, A., Hirsch, E., Arzimanoglou, A., Genton, P., Motte, J., de Saint Martin, A., Valenti, M.P., Boulay, C., De Bellescize, J., Kéo-Kosal, P., Boutry-Kryza, N., Edery, P., Sanlaville, D., Szepetowski, P., 2012. Epileptic encephalopathies of the Landau-Kleffner and continuous spike and waves during slow-wave sleep types: genomic dissection makes the link with autism. Epilepsia 53 (9), 1526–1538.

Meletti, S., Ruggieri, A., Avanzini, P., Caramaschi, E., Filippini, M., Bergonzini, P., Monti, G., Vignoli, A., Olivotto, S., Mastrangelo, M., Santucci, M., Gobbi, G., Veggiotti, P., Vaudano, A.E., 2016. Extrastriate visual cortex in idiopathic occipital epilepsies: the contribution of retinotopic areas to spike generation. Epilepsia 57 (6), 896–906.

Monteiro, J.P., Roulet-Perez, E., Davidoff, V., Deonna, T., 2001. Primary neonatal thalamic haemorrhage and epilepsy with continuous spike-wave during sleep: a longitudinal follow-up of a possible significant relation. Eur. J. Paediatr. Neurol. 5 (1), 41–47.

Nobili, L., Ferrillo, F., Baglietto, M.G., Beelke, M., De Carli, F., De Negri, E., Schiavi, G., Rosadini, G., De Negri, M., 1999. Relationship of sleep interictal epileptiform discharges to sigma activity (12-16 Hz) in benign epilepsy of childhood with rolandic spikes. Clin. Neurophysiol. 110 (1), 39–46.

Nobili, L., Baglietto, M.G., Beelke, M., De Carli, F., De Negri, E., Gaggero, R., Rosadini, G., Veneselli, E., Ferrillo, F., 2001. Distribution of epileptiform discharges during nREM sleep in the CSWSS syndrome: relationship with sigma and delta activities. Epilepsy Res. 44 (2–3), 119–128.

Nobili, L., Baglietto, M.G., Beelke, M., De Carli, F., De Negri, E., Tortorelli, S., Ferrillo, F., 2000. Spindles-inducing mechanism modulates sleep activation of interictal epileptiform discharges in the Landau-Kleffner syndrome. Epilepsia 41 (2), 201–206.

Panayiotopoulos, C.P., 1999. Benign Childhood Partial Seizures and Related Epileptic Syndromes. John Libbey & Company Ltd, London.

Panayiotopoulos, C.P., 2002. Panayiotopoulos Syndrome: A Common and Benign Childhood Epileptic Syndrome. John Libbey & Company, London.

Panayiotopoulos, C.P., Michael, M., Sanders, S., Valeta, T., Koutroumanidis, M., 2008. Benign childhood focal epilepsies: assessment of established and newly recognized syndromes. Brain 131 (Pt 9) , 2264–2286.

Patry, G., Lyagoubi, S., Tassinari, C.A., 1971. Subclinical electrical status epilepticus induced by sleep in children. Arch. Neurol. 24, 242–252.

Quigg, M., Noachtar, S., 2012. Sleep-potentiated epileptic discharges, language regression, and pediatric thalamic lesions. Neurology 78 (22), 1708–1709.

Reutlinger, C., Helbig, I., Gawelczyk, B., Subero, J.I., Tönnies, H., et al., 2010. Deletions in 16p13 including GRIN2A in patients with intellectual disability, various dysmorphic features, and seizure disorders of the rolandic region. Epilepsia 51 (9), 1870–1873.

Rudolf, G., Valenti, M.P., Hirsch, E., Szepetowski, P., 2009. From rolandic epilepsy to continuous spike-and-waves during sleep and Landau-Kleffner syndromes: insights into possible genetic factors. Epilepsia 50 (Suppl. 7), 25–28.

Saltik, S., Uluduz, D., Cokar, O., Demirbilek, V., Dervent, A., 2005. A clinical and EEG study on idiopathic partial epilepsies with evolution into ESES spectrum disorders. Epilepsia 46 (4), 524–533.

Sánchez Fernández, I., Loddenkemper, T., Peters, J.M., Kothare, S.V., 2012. Electrical status epilepticus in sleep: clinical presentation and pathophysiology. Pediatr. Neurol. 47 (6), 390–410.

Sanchez Fernandez, I., Loddenkemper, T., 2012. Pediatric focal epilepsy syndromes. J. Clin. Neurophysiol. 29 (5), 425–440.

Tassinari, C.A., Dravet, C., Roger, J., 1977. Encephalopathy related to electrical status epilepticus during slow sleep. Electroencephalogr. Clin. Neurophysiol. 43, 529–530.

Tassinari, C.A., Rubboli, G., Volpi, L., Meletti, S., d'Orsi, G., Franca, M., Sabetta, A.R., Riguzzi, P., Gardella, E., Zaniboni, A., Michelucci, R., 2000. Encephalopathy with electrical status epilepticus during slow sleep or ESES syndrome including the acquired aphasia. Clin. Neurophysiol. 111 (Suppl. 2), S94–S102.

Taylor, I., Berkovic, S.F., Kivity, S., Scheffer, I.E., 2008. Benign occipital epilepsies of childhood: clinical features and genetics. Brain 131, 2287–2294.

Teixeira, K.C., Montenegro, M.A., Cendes, F., Guimarães, C.A., Guerreiro, C.A., Guerreiro, M.M., 2007. Clinical and electroencephalographic features of patients with polymicrogyria. J. Clin. Neurophysiol. 24, 244–251.

Terzano, M.G., Parrino, L., Spaggiari, M.C., Barusi, R., Simeoni, S., 1991. Discriminatory effect of cyclic alternating pattern in focal lesional and benign rolandic interictal spikes during sleep. Epilepsia 32 (5), 616–628.

Tükel, K., Jasper, H., 1952. The electroencephalogram in parasagittal lesions. Electroencephalogr. Clin. Neurophysiol. 4 (4), 481–494.

Vannest, J., Tenney, J.R., Gelineau-Morel, R., Maloney, T., Glauser, T.A., 2015. Cognitive and behavioral outcomes in benign childhood epilepsy with centrotemporal spikes. Epilepsy Behav. 45, 85–91.

Veggiotti, P., Beccaria, F., Guerrini, R., Capovilla, G., Lanzi, G., 1999. Continuous spike-and-wave activity during slow-wave sleep: syndrome or EEG pattern? Epilepsia 40, 1593–1601.

Verrotti, A., Matricardi, S., Di Giacomo, D.L., Rapino, D., Chiarelli, F., Coppola, G., 2013. Neuropsychological impairment in children with Rolandic epilepsy and in their siblings. Epilepsy Behav. 28 (1), 108–112.

Wong, P.K., 1991. Source modelling of the rolandic focus. Brain Topogr. 4 (2), 105–112.

Yoshinaga, H., Koutroumanidis, M., Kobayashi, K., Shirasawa, A., Kikumoto, K., Inoue, T., Oka, M., Ohtsuka, Y., 2006. EEG dipole characteristics in Panayiotopoulos syndrome. Epilepsia 47 (4), 781–787.

7

Epileptic Encephalopathies

Epileptic encephalopathies (EEs) constitute a contradictory, however widely used, category in epileptology recognized by the International League Against Epilepsy. EEs are epilepsy-related conditions of early-damaged large systems of the brain, presumably involving the corticothalamic system. The main criterion is that the associated cognitive symptoms are caused by epilepsy itself; in other words, the effects of those factors causing the epilepsy as well as of the applied antiepileptic drugs need to be excluded. Structural changes and neurology signs may be associated but are not essential. The concept of system epilepsies overlaps with EEs (Capovilla et al., 2013).

The weakness of the EE category has been considered, blurring the actual mechanisms linking cognitive decline to epilepsy (Jehi et al., 2015; Howell et al., 2016).

There is a conceptual difference between EEs and encephalopathies with epilepsy. In the latter group there is a common cause, e.g., tuberous sclerosis, underlying both epilepsy and the cognitive symptoms, whereas in electrical status epilepticus in sleep (ESES) belonging to the EEs, it is likely that the sleep-related interictal discharges and seizures themselves cause the cognitive deficit.

EEs typically start in infancy or early childhood. They are characterized by an active EEG with abundant interictal signs not related to a single focus, occurring dominantly in, or activated by, slow-wave sleep (SWS). The specific combination of symptoms constituting different EEs might be due to a common pathomechanism related to variable etiologic factors. Some EEs may have a genetic background; most of them are not yet clarified. There is a progression to the full-blown picture in most cases, which may become stagnant and resistant to treatment after.

The pathomechanism of cognitive impairment is supposed to be caused by the interference of the abundant interictal and ictal discharges with the widespread corticothalamic network functions, having a major impact in fueling the activity of the associative neocortex [see Blume, 2001, for Lennox–Gastaut syndrome (LGS)]. Here the epileptic disorder is usually very early and is assumed to take over the organization of physiological networks. For understanding the two steps in the evolution of EEs, the term "developmental" has been proposed (Scheffer et al., 2017) for those encephalopathies with a developmental component, naming them "developmental epileptic encephalopathies."

In addition to the epileptic macrodischarges, an abundance of pathological high-frequency ripples is characteristic, seeming to have a forecasting significance (Kobayashi et al., 2011, 2015) for EEs. The pathological high-frequency oscillation vastly increases in non–rapid eye movement sleep (Staba, 2012). Owing to technical progress, these pathological ripple discharges are more and more detectable not only by intracranial electrodes, but by scalp leads as well.

Pathological high-frequency oscillations (HFOs; fast ripples with 250- to 500-Hz frequencies) have been described in most childhood EEs. In infantile EEs with burst-suppression activity (Ohtahara syndrome and early myoclonic encephalopathy), Toda et al. (2015) reported on bilateral parietooccipital dominant 80- to 150-Hz frequency ripples during bursts, not detected in controls, by digital EEGs sampled at 500 Hz. Endoh et al. (2011) detected 10- to 20-Hz activity in 1- to 2-s runs over the posterior regions of the skull in 12 of 68 infants carrying different prenatal and perinatal lesions. West syndrome developed 4–5 months later in 9 of the 12 infants.

Kobayashi et al. (2004), performing scalp EEGs, detected 50- to 100-Hz ictal fast activity spells during 345 infantile spasms of 11 infants. The fast activity was mainly bilateral. Kobayashi et al. (2015) recorded 1519 interictal fast oscillations during the sleep of 17 infants suffering from West syndrome. The frequency ranges of the oscillations fell between 40 and 150 Hz (median 56.6) and their occurrence was 24–171/min (median 66). They supposed that the pathological fast oscillations interfered with cognitive functions.

HFOs recorded with scalp EEG in rolandic epilepsy ($N = 32$) and in Panayiotopoulos syndrome ($N = 13$) were reported by the same group in 2011. The fast frequency ranged between 93.8 and 152.3 Hz and was joined to spikes in 71.3% (Kobayashi et al., 2011). The frequency of the oscillations showed a statistically significant negative correlation with the distance from the prior seizure. The fast oscillations were associated in time with ESES and were much more prominent than in those subjects without ESES, suggesting a prognostic significance.

Kobayashi et al. (2010) scrutinized HFOs in ESES. Ten children ages 6–9 years were examined; three of them suffered from Landau–Kleffner syndrome (LKS). The authors registered fast oscillations of 97.7–140.6 Hz frequency and supposed the oscillations' interference with cognitive functions.

The presence of HFO activity correlating with the severity and progression of EEs supports the impact of HFO activity on the cognitive impairment in EEs as well. The cutoff frequencies of normal and pathological HFO activity in infants and children are not yet clear.

The types of EEs are the following: early infantile EE or early infantile EE with burst-suppression pattern (its prototype is Ohtahara syndrome), West syndrome, LGS, LKS, and ESES (see in Chapter 6).

EARLY INFANTILE EPILEPTIC ENCEPHALOPATHY WITH BURST-SUPPRESSION PATTERN

This syndrome is characterized by a burst-suppression activity seen on the EEG of children under age 3 years. Polyspike–wave bursts and suppression of electrical activity alternate during both wakefulness and sleep, mainly during sleep. The bursts are generally symmetrical, but not always synchronous over the two hemispheres. If there is a lesional hemisphere containing a brain defect like a hemimegalencephaly, a cortical dysplasia, or schizencephaly, it dominates the EEG syndrome. Structural brain abnormalities make the majority of early infantile EEs, although metabolic disorders make an important etiologic group. Nonketotic hyperglycinemia is the most frequent; pyridoxine deficiency, disturbance of carnitine turnover, or Leigh disease occur as well.

The two main forms are hard to differentiate: (1) early myoclonic encephalopathy with myocloni linked to EEG bursts mainly during night sleep and (2) Ohtahara syndrome (Ohtahara et al., 1987), characterized by tonic spasms. The syndrome may progress to West syndrome.

WEST SYNDROME

This syndrome occurs in infants ages 3–12 months. Three basic features have originally been described: (1) EEG hypsarrhythmia; (2) infantile spasms—numberless full-body axial jerks typically after awakening, temporal and other motor seizures may present as well; and (3) a severe cognitive decline. The introduction of vigabatrin has improved the prognosis, abolishing the criterion of cognitive decline. This is a good example of cognitive symptoms caused by epilepsy itself and helped by antiepileptic treatment.

The EEG hypsarrhythmia may turn to a burst-suppression pattern during sleep or even during wakefulness, especially in severe cases. This may be unilateral in the presence of brain damage, affecting the damaged hemisphere only.

Of the underlying structural lesions, tuberous sclerosis is the most frequent. Other etiologies like hemimegalencephaly, lissencephaly, cortical dysplasia, Sturge–Weber syndrome, or perinatal hypoxia, as well as genetic factors, may underlie the condition. Ohtahara syndrome can progress to West syndrome and later to LGS, providing an example of a disease spectrum.

There are cases with and without a structural brain lesion. Seizure semiology and EEG may manifest focal features in the lesional group, whereas the symptoms are symmetrical in nonlesional cases.

West syndrome is an age-specific reaction type; i.e., in a certain age window diverse etiologic factors create a relatively uniform combination of symptoms.

The burst-suppression EEG pattern seen also in early EE represents the "all or nothing law" type of cortical excitability cycle. The burst discharges make a great metabolic demand on the cortex resulting in a "full" exhaustion, reflected by a temporary suppression of cortical activity. The regeneration is followed by a burst-like state of excitability resulting in synchronous nondifferentiated intensive discharges and then a phase of exhaustion again. The spasms associate with a secondary synchronization with preserved hemispheric asymmetry. Hypsarrhythmia and infantile spasms are consistent with the actual maturity level of the brain, not necessarily interrelated (after the vanishing of hypsarrhythmia, the spasms may persist). Some months after the onset of West syndrome, and in connection with the maturation of the brain, it may turn into a focal or polyfocal epilepsy or LGS.

Chugani et al. (1992) in Detroit analyzed the neuroimaging (MRI, PET) features of West syndrome, and they could provide data on the neuronal networks involved. Typically, they found a cortical dysplasia, generating focal/regional epileptic activity. The focal malformation could generally be revealed just by PET studies owing to myelination features (not yet myelinated) of the age group. There was a symmetrical hypermetabolism of the lenticular nuclei irrespective of the presence or absence of cortical dysplasia. The data suggested a network between the cortical (dysgenic) focus, the brain stem, and the lenticular nuclei. They hypothesized that in a critical age window, this

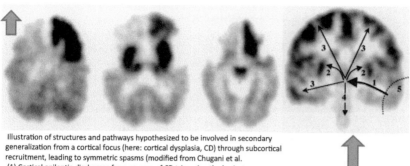

Illustration of structures and pathways hypothesized to be involved in secondary generalization from a cortical focus (here: cortical dysplasia, CD) through subcortical recruitment, leading to symmetric spasms (modified from Chugani et al. (1) Cortical epileptic discharges from an area of CD triggering the brainstem, presumably the dorsal raphe area, a brain region with a large number of serotonergic cell bodies. (2) Bilateral, serotonergic raphe-striatal projections activate the striatum. (3) Raphe-cortical interactions induce hypsarrhythmia on the EEG. (4) Propagation to the spinal cord can lead to symmetric spasms. (5) Surgical resection of the primary offending lesion (the area of CD) stops the circuit from being activated.

FIGURE 7.1   Hypermetabolism of the left frontal cortex and bilateral symmetrical hypermetabolism of the lenticular nuclei and the brain stem in a patient with intractable infantile spasms. Chugani et al. (1992) worked out a hypothesis to explain the unilateral lesional origin with bilateral electroclinical epileptic manifestations in West syndrome. They assumed that the pathological impulses from a cortical dysplasia trigger the brain stem, presumably the dorsal raphe area serotoninergic neurons. The bilateral raphe–striatal projections activate the striatum, thereby inducing hypsarrhythmia on the scalp. The excision of the focal lesion (dysplastic cortex) stops the activation of the circuits.

network activity may produce secondary generalization leading to the bilateral spasms (Fig. 7.1). The surgical removal of the primary epileptogenic cortical region could successfully stop bilateral spasms in some of the patients.

LENNOX–GASTAUT SYNDROME

LGS starts typically at ages 3–5 years, under age 8 in most cases. A later onset above age 10 years occurs; it is called late LGS (Stenzel and Panteli, 1981).

The syndrome may present "out of the blue" in many patients, but in an important group of children it is preceded by West syndrome. It appears in children with cognitive impairment in more than 50%. In 20%–30% of them brain imaging may reveal some structural abnormalities, or only the cognitive deficit indicates the impairment. Several types of seizures may occur; tonic seizures are the most typical. Generalized tonic–clonic seizures are infrequent; atonic seizures and atypical absences appear frequently. The incidence of a status epilepticus is high compared to the rest of EEs, sadly contributing to the progression of the syndrome.

There are several types of EEG features in LGS: (1) Bilateral synchronous, frontal dominant slow (1.5–2.5 Hz) spike–waves emerge from a slow background activity. The spike–waves are not photosensible and do not react much to hyperventilation. They are importantly activated by SWS,

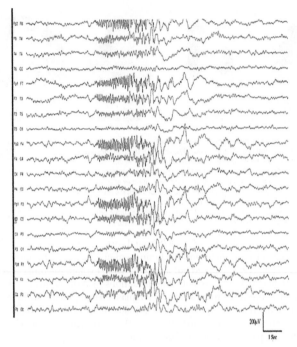

FIGURE 7.2   Examples of generalized paroxysmal fast activity with no Lennox–Gastaut syndrome and no cognitive impairment.

sometimes covering half of its duration. (2) In deep SWS, bilateral synchronous alpha-frequency or more rapid runs, called generalized paroxysmal fast activity (GPFA), occur, lasting for a few seconds and followed by exhaustion (Fig. 7.2). GPFA rarely occurs during wakefulness, and never in rapid eye movement sleep. It can be evoked by sound and other sensory stimulation applied during SWS. It is consistent with mini-seizure activity, suggested by the associated tonic axial clinical attacks, e.g., an increase in the patient's muscle tone (generally in the neck) and eye opening.

In LGS, there is a poor response to traditional antiepileptic drugs; no durable seizure freedom is achieved.

Late LGS emerges through a secondary generalization process from difficult-to-treat temporal or frontal epilepsies (Halász, 1991).

LGS as a distinct syndrome has been challenged for several reasons. First, GPFA is also seen in difficult-to-treat idiopathic generalized epilepsies with no cognitive impairment (Halász et al., 2004) (Fig. 7.2). Second, an iatrogenic origin of GPFA is possible, given its more frequent occurrence after a long-term benzodiazepine and barbiturate treatment than without (Halász, 1991). The LGS-related EEG patterns have been analyzed with modern neuroimaging methods (Archer et al., 2014). EEG–functional MRI (fMRI) studies have been performed in six LGS patients during slow spike–wave discharges and GPFA episodes. During GPFA episodes, an important signal increase occurred in the frontal and parietal association cortices, the thalamus, the pons, and the default mode network. During slow spike–waves, there was a prior signal increase in the thalamus and the association cortex and an important signal decrease following the discharge. These features disappeared after successful lesionectomy, resulting in seizure freedom. There were no specific changes in the primary cortex. The EEG–fMRI results suggest that the networks visualized during the two basic patterns produce secondary epileptic networks constituting the LGS phenotype. The understanding of secondary networks is different from that of secondary bilateral synchrony. According to the secondary network concept, there is a permanent interictal epileptic distortion with no direct impact on seizure generation. (This contradicts the occurrence of the small tonic seizures associated with GPFA.) Thus, whereas the interictal networks do not have a seizure-generating activity, they may have an impact on several important symptoms, e.g., cognitive impairment.

LANDAU–KLEFFNER SYNDROME: ACQUIRED EPILEPTIC APHASIA WITH REGIONAL ESES-LIKE SLEEP ACTIVATION

Acquired epileptic aphasia starting with acoustic agnosia and word deafness was described by Landau and Kleffner in 1957.

After many doubts and contradictions, it is now clear that in some subgroups of the idiopathic focal childhood epilepsies, e.g., in atypical rolandic epilepsy and Panayiotopoulos syndrome, a speech disturbance may evolve at ages 2–7 years, with an important activation of spike discharges during SWS over the temporal lobes, more so on the dominant side (Deonna and Roulet-Perez, 2010). The speech disturbance is mainly consistent with an auditory dysphasia, but additional mental changes, e.g., autism and psychosis-like events, may present as well. The link of cognitive symptoms with sleep EEG discharges could be but slowly clarified, possibly because of the variable disease course and the lack of longitudinal follow-up studies. PET and fMRI studies have shown a link between the patterns of cognitive loss and the topography of EEG discharges (Tassinari et al., 2009). The age curve of cognitive and EEG symptoms parallels idiopathic childhood epilepsies. The malignant turn of the disease generally occurs on the basis of an atypical rolandic epilepsy or Panayiotopoulos syndrome. About half of the cases are underlain by a structural brain lesion. The cognitive symptoms might be reversible if LKS is diagnosed in time, sometimes responding to corticosteroid treatment. In the rolandic epilepsy–LKS spectrum there are patients suffering from just mild and transient disturbance of speech, whereas others with a persisting oromotor deficit (anterior opercular syndrome) may recover later, similar to LKS. Familial cases with siblings suffering from LKS or rolandic epilepsy have been described.

Based on these data LKS is considered a malignant variant of the perisylvian epilepsy spectrum diseases with an augmented regional ESES occurring over the posterior speech regions of the dominant hemisphere (see also Chapter 6) (Halász et al., 2005).

Genetic findings support the idea of a spectrum disease continuum involving rolandic epilepsy (and Panayiotopoulos syndrome), atypical rolandic epilepsy, LKS, and ESES (Rudolf et al., 2009; Lesca et al., 2012; Lemke et al., 2013).

The common features of EEs are as follows:

- Most of them are age related, starting in early childhood, in the phase of high brain plasticity.
- The same combination of symptoms may be generated by different etiologies contributed to by genetic factors.
- The cognitive dysfunction is supposed to be underlain by the disordered association cortex.
- A pathological HFO (fast ripples) is present in all forms during sleep.
- The interictal epileptic activity has a more important negative impact than the seizures themselves. It is possible that the cognitive impairment of EEs has a mechanism similar to that of ESES: abundant interictal spiking and pathological ripple activity during sleep, and interictal epileptic discharges (IEDs) and HFO activity interfering with sleep plastic functions (Fig. 7.3). The impairment might be more severe in EEs, compared to ESES and LKS, because of the much younger age at disease onset.

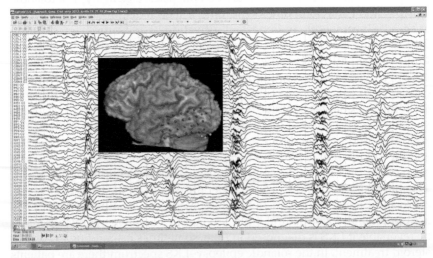

FIGURE 7.3 Epileptic encephalopathy with focal features explored by implanted subdural electrodes (corticography: slow spike–wave discharges conjoined by high-frequency oscillation ripples). *Inset*: The territory of the cortex from where the activity was recorded is covered by grid electrodes.

THE COMMON PATHOMECHANISM OF COGNITIVE IMPAIRMENT IN CHILDHOOD EPILEPTIC ENCEPHALOPATHIES WITH IMPORTANT SLEEP ACTIVATION WITH INTERICTAL EPILEPTIC DISCHARGES AND HIGH-FREQUENCY OSCILLATIONS

Childhood EEs share the feature of abundant interictal activity during SWS.

The burst-suppression activity covering the whole sleep in early neonatal encephalopathies probably interferes with normal brain development.

In West syndrome, sleep is disfigured by hypsarrhythmia or by its modified variant, alternating with burst-suppression activity. The same or even worse cognitive effect holds true for the cognitive impact of this pattern, also due to the additional frequent, variable-topography seizures. The cognitive harm caused by hypsarrhythmia and frequent infantile spasms is confirmed by the cognitive improvement on vigabatrin, treating epileptic activity.

In LGS, the abundant diffuse slow spike–waves and GPFA with or without tonic seizures may interfere with normal cognitive functioning.

During the transformation process of idiopathic hyperexcitability conditions to ESES, it is well known that the cognitive decline of the affected children clearly follows the enormous activation—abundance, synchronization, and propagation—of spikes during sleep.

In ESES, an important part of SWS is covered by epileptic discharges. It has been shown that these discharges interfere with the normal downscaling of slow waves during night sleep (Bölsterli et al., 2011; Cantalupo et al., 2011; Bigna et al., 2014), compromising the plastic processes.

The harmfulness of IEDs was raised by Colin Binnie, who demonstrated the instant cognitive interference (transient cognitive impairment, or TCI) of centrotemporal spikes of rolandic epilepsy and bilateral spike–wave paroxysms of idiopathic generalized epilepsy patients (Binnie, 1996). This finding made clinicians wonder that the frequent spiking in focal childhood epilepsies may need pharmacotherapy to prevent cognitive decline. The reasoning underlying this idea was that the observed cognitive symptoms in rolandic epilepsy were considered the consequences of spiking (however, centrotemporal spiking is present also in the relatives of rolandic patients who never had seizures nor cognitive decline). The clinical research on the TCI phenomenon had serious limitations. First, the cognitive impairment was measured only instantly at the time of an electrical interictal event, and second, the temporal (hippocampal) spiking of medial temporal lobe epilepsy patients and epileptic encephalopathic children known to be candidates for chronic cognitive (especially memory) decay has never been investigated.

Taking into consideration these findings obviously related to genetic factors in epileptic and nonepileptic subjects, we view these EEG features as endophenotypic traits not necessarily linked with epilepsy (Fig. 6.5 of Chapter 6). What is the difference between "red" (related to epilepsy or cognitive impairment) and "green" (with no harm) spikes? The answer to this question has arrived from the studies linking IEDs and pathological HFOs (fast ripples). van Klink et al. (2016) showed the concomitance of HFOs with "red" spikes of rolandic epilepsy children, unlike the "green" spikes of children without seizures. Moreover, HFO activity was more intense (based on several parameters) in those children who suffered the malignant transformation toward ESES. The HFO activity therefore seems indeed a more faithful surrogate marker of epileptogenicity than spikes.

Another aspect of the IED-related cognitive impairment research field is that we need a switch from dealing with "transient" to "long-term" (and possibly progressive) cognitive impairment. Performing long-term cognitive studies and sleep studies is hard, requiring highly organized cooperative work continuously embracing decades.

The research linking epilepsy to network activities considers interictal and ictal conditions as different network states. Ictal states represent pathological peaks of activity, expressed in episodic changes of behavior, whereas the interictal states constitute a more continuous background of the disorder. The influence of this hidden ongoing and insidious interictal activity manifesting no spectacular events has remained more or less unknown even after so many years of intensive epilepsy research.

References

Archer, J.S., Warren, A.E., Jackson, G.D., Abbott, D.F., 2014. Conceptualizing Lennox–Gastaut syndrome as a secondary network epilepsy. Front. Neurol. 5, 225.

Bigna, K., Bölsterli, H., Fattinger, S., Kurth, S., LeBourgeois, M.K., et al., 2014. Spike wave location and density disturb sleep slow waves in patients with CSWS (continuous spike waves during sleep). Epilepsia 55 (4), 584–591.

Binnie, C.D., 1996. Cognitive effects of subclinical EEG discharges. Neurophysiol. Clin. 26 (3), 138–142.

Blume, W.T., 2001. Pathogenesis of Lennox–Gastaut syndrome: considerations and hypotheses. Epileptic Disord. 3 (4), 183–196.

Bölsterli, B.K., Schmitt, B., Bast, T., Critelli, H., Heinzle, J., Jenni, O.G., Huber, R., 2011. Impaired slow wave sleep downscaling in encephalopathy with status epilepticus during sleep (ESES). Clin. Neurophysiol. 122 (9), 1779–1787.

Cantalupo, G., Rubboli, G., Tassinari, C.A., 2011. Night-time unravelling of the brain web: impaired synaptic downscaling in ESES-the Penelope syndrome. Clin. Neurophysiol. 122 (9), 1691–1692.

Capovilla, G., Moshé, S.L., Wolf, P., Avanzini, G., 2013. Epileptic encephalopathy as models of system epilepsy. Epilepsia 8 (Suppl. 54), 34–37.

Chugani, H.T., Shewmon, D.A., Sankar, R., Chen, B.C., Phelps, M.E., 1992. Infantile spasms: II. Lenticular nuclei and brain stem activation on positron emission tomography. Ann. Neurol. 31 (2), 212–219.

Deonna, T., Roulet-Perez, E., 2010. Early-onset acquired epileptic aphasia (Landau–Kleffner syndrome, LKS) and regressive autistic disorders with epileptic EEG abnormalities: the continuing debate. Brain Dev. 32 (9), 746–752.

Endoh, F., Yoshinaga, H., Ishizaki, Y., Oka, M., Kobayashi, K., Ohtsuka, Y., 2011. Abnormal fast activity before the onset of west syndrome. Neuropediatrics 42 (2), 51–54.

Halász, P., Janszky, J., Barcs, G., Szűcs, A., 2004. Generalised paroxysmal fast activity (GPFA) is not always a sign of malignant epileptic encephalopathy. Seizure 13 (4), 270–276.

Halász, P., 1991. Runs of rapid spikes in sleep: a characteristic EEG expression of generalized malignant epileptic encephalopathies, a conceptual review with new pharmacological data. Epilepsy Res. Suppl. 2, 49–71.

Halász, P., Kelemen, A., Clemens, B., Saracz, J., Rosdy, B., Rásonyi, G., Szűcs, A., 2005. The perisylvian epileptic network. A unifying concept. Ideggyogy. Sz. 2005 58 (1–2), 21–31.

Howell, K.B., Harvey, A.S., Archer, J.S., 2016. Epileptic encephalopathy: use and misuse of a clinically and conceptually important concept. Epilepsia 57 (3).

Jehi, L., Wyllie, E., Devinsky, O., 2015. Epileptic encephalopathies: optimizing seizure control and developmental outcome. Epilepsia 56 (10), 1486–1489.

Kobayashi, K., Oka, M., Akiyama, T., Inoue, T., Abiru, K., Ogino, T., Yoshinaga, H., Ohtsuka, Y., Oka, E., 2004. Very fast rhythmic activity on scalp EEG associated with epileptic spasms. Epilepsia 45 (5), 488–496.

Kobayashi, K., Akiyama, T., Oka, M., Endoh, F., Yoshinaga, H., 2015. A storm of fast (40–150Hz) oscillations during hypsarrhythmia in west syndrome. Ann. Neurol. 77 (1), 58–67.

Kobayashi, K., Watanabe, Y., Inoue, T., Oka, M., Yoshinaga, H., Ohtsuka, Y., 2010. Scalp-recorded high-frequency oscillations in childhood sleep-induced electrical status epilepticus. Epilepsia 51 (10), 2190–2194.

Kobayashi, K., Yoshinaga, H., Toda, Y., Inoue, T., Oka, M., 2011. High-frequency oscillations in idiopathic partial epilepsy of childhood. Epilepsia 52 (10), 1812–1819.

Landau, W.M., Kleffner, F.R., 1957. Syndrome of acquired aphasia with convulsive disorder in children. Neurology 7 (8), 523–530.

Lemke, J.R., Lal, D., Reinthaler, E.M., Steiner, I., Nothnagel, M., 2013. Mutations in GRIN2A cause idiopathic focal epilepsy with rolandic spikes. Nat. Genet. 45 (9), 1067–1072.

Lesca, G., Rudolf, G., Labalme, A., Hirsch, E., Arzimanoglou, A., et al., 2012. Epileptic encephalopathies of the Landau–Kleffner and continuous spike and waves during slow-wave sleep types: genomic dissection makes the link with autism. Epilepsia 53 (9), 1526–1538.

Ohtahara, S., Ohtsuka, Y., Yamatogi, Y., Oka, E., 1987. The early-infantile epileptic encephalopathy with suppression-burst: developmental aspects. Brain Dev. 9 (4), 371–376.

Rudolf, G., Valenti, M.P., Hirsch, E., Szepetowski, P., 2009. From rolandic epilepsy to continuous spike-and-waves during sleep and Landau-Kleffner syndromes: insights into possible genetic factors. Epilepsia 50, (Suppl. 7), 25–28.

Scheffer, I.E., Berkovic, S., Capovilla, G., Connolly, M.B., French, J., Guilhoto, L., Hirsch, E., Jain, S., Mathern, G.W., Moshé, S.L., Nordli, D.R., Perucca, E., Tomson, T., Wiebe, S., Zhang, Y.H., Zuberi, S.M., 2017. ILAE classification of the epilepsies: position paper of the ILAE commission for classification and terminology. Epilepsia 58 (4), 512–521.

Staba, R.J., 2012. Normal and pathologic high-frequency oscillations. In: Jasper's Basic Mechanisms of the Epilepsies [Internet], fourth edition. National Center for Biotechnology Information (US), Bethesda (MD).

Stenzel, E., Panteli, C., 1981. Lennox–Gastaut-Syndrom des 2. Lebensjahrzehntes. In: Hemschmidt, H., Rentz, R., Jungmann, J. (Eds.), Epilepsie. Thieme, Stuttgart, pp. 99–107.

Tassinari, C.A., Cantalupo, G., Rios-Pohl, L., Giustina, E.D., Rubboli, G., 2009. Encephalopathy with status epilepticus during slow sleep: "the Penelope syndrome". Epilepsia 50 (Suppl. 7), 4–8.

Toda, Y., Kobayashi, K., Hayashi, Y., Inoue, T., Oka, M., Endo, F., Yoshinaga, H., Ohtsuka, Y., 2015. High-frequency EEG activity in epileptic encephalopathy with suppression-burst. Brain Dev. 37 (2), 230–236.

van Klink, N.E.C., van't Klooster, M.A., Leijten, F.S.S., Jacobs, J., Braun, K.P.J., Zijlmans, July 2016. Ripples on Rolandic spikes: a marker of epilepsy severity. In: Proceedings of 2nd International workshop on HFO in epilepsy Freiburg im Bresgau Epilepsia, vol. 57(7), pp. 1179–1189.

Summary

In this book, we aimed to give an overview of the important links between non–rapid eye movement (NREM) sleep and epilepsy armed by the results of contemporary sleep research.

We discussed the interrelationship of epilepsy and sleep in those major epilepsies with a characteristic relationship with NREM sleep and tried to reinterpret them as system epilepsies. System epilepsy is an increasingly accepted concept considering epileptic networks as the occupants of the affected brain systems, distorting their development and function. Owing to this specific network invasion, the epileptic manifestations are closely interwoven with system functions: they are ignited by the activation of the system or interfere with its functioning.

We have shown that major epilepsies can be interpreted as exaggerations of cerebral plasticity in the corticothalamic and hippocampal structures. Their epileptic derailment and consequent malformed function result in distorted plasticity, i.e., cognitive impairment.

We have described here:

absence epilepsy as a sleep-system epilepsy ignited by shifts toward NREM sleep due to the epileptic invasion of the corticothalamic system's burst-firing mode;

nocturnal frontal lobe epilepsy as a system epilepsy of arousal and alarm from NREM sleep (paralleling the nonepileptic variants, the arousal parasomnias);

juvenile myoclonic epilepsy (Janz syndrome) and reading epilepsy as related variations, both system epilepsies of the corticothalamic motor and cognitive frontal subsystems;

medial temporal lobe epilepsy as a system epilepsy of the declarative memory system based on an epileptic distortion of the hippocampal and hippocampofrontal memory consolidation system;

age-dependent idiopathic childhood regional hyperexcitability conditions (HIECs) such as rolandic epilepsy and Panayiotopoulos syndrome, system epilepsies of the perisylvian epileptic network;

electrical status epilepticus in sleep [ESES when global; Landau–
Kleffner syndrome (LKS) when partial], representing extremes
(exaggerations) of the spectrum of HIEC sleep activation;
epileptic developmental encephalopathies.

Three main ways to cognitive impairment have been recognized:

1. the epileptic transformation of the corticothalamic system
   a. involving variable bilateral sectors in ESES interfering with the
      downscaling of slow waves and synaptic activity
   b. constantly involving the dominant hemisphere's posterior part in
      LKS
2. the interference of spiking with memory consolidation in medial
   temporal lobe epilepsy (obstructing the nightly upscaling of memory-
   specific, mainly frontal synaptic functions)

We have emphasized the special role of sleep in the activation of interictal discharges (with and without clinical seizures) in the form of spikes
and high-frequency oscillations leading to the development of chronic
cognitive decline.

We see two types of the interrelationship between sleep and epilepsy,
with or without cognitive consequences. In the first type (HIEC-ESES/
LKS, MTLE) the epileptic activation interferes with certain cognitive functions during sleep, and in the second (AE, NFLE) the sleep/arousal system
is penetrated by epilepsy, which is ignited during falling asleep or arousal.
The first type is mainly associated with IEDs and cognitive decline,
whereas, in the second type, there are outstanding seizures without IEDs
and cognitive decline. These patterns suggest that interictal spiking during NREM sleep should be a decisive factor in cognitive impairment in
sleep-related epilepsies. This emerging conclusion points to the need to
bring interictal discharges (together with the related HFO) into the focus
of further research about cognitive impairment in epilepsies. This will be
very difficult due to two basic obstacles. Firstly, our oldest and more pain-
ful "Achilles heel" in the treatment of epilepsies is that antiepileptic drugs
have no effect on epilepsy itself; they fight only seizures and the "peaks"
of the disease and leave the background pathology untouched. Secondly,
it is not the spikes themselves that cause the cognitive harm; rather it is
their interference with the plastic sleep function. One solution would be
to find effective treatment against IEDs, or find effective treatment against
IEDs; the other one would be a way to recover or substitute sleep slow
oscillation. For the latter is being tried by transcranial magnetic stimulation or boosting sleep functions with acoustic stimulation (see Ngo et al.,
2013, Bellesi et al., 2014 in references of Chapter 1).

The link between sleep and epilepsy is a unique merger including three
amalgamated steps. (1) NREM sleep activates epilepsy, creating templates

in both the corticothalamic and the hippocampal system functions for epileptic exaggeration; (2) the epileptic network manifestations are amplified and synchronized during NREM sleep; (3) interictal epileptic discharges interfere with sleep plastic functions (memory consolidation and refreshing the synaptic capacity to learn). We can also say that epileptic discharges are excessive (exaggerated) copies of the communication signals, obstructing cognitive functioning. The cognitive malfunction is not the direct effect of epileptic activity, but rather of the interference with sleep plastic changes. In the witty words of Steriade, "epilepsy and sleep are bedfellows," and we can add that this clasp between sleep and epilepsy during NREM sleep has deadly consequences for our most important human faculties: memory and learning.

In reviewing the large landscape of epilepsies, we tried to use the results of the new structural and functional neuroimaging methods to find and specify the places and roles of the players in the epileptic process, like ictal and interictal manifestations and high-frequency oscillations.

The research on the interrelationship of sleep and epilepsy has opened new vistas with important heuristic significance. From the practical side we are emphasizing the need to incorporate sleep studies into the evaluation of epileptic patients. Theoretically, we need to have more insight into the dark side of epilepsy hidden in sleep. Clinical sleep studies can be the litmus paper unmasking them.

Index

'*Note*: Page numbers followed by "f" indicate figures and "t" indicate tables.'

Printed and bound by CPI Group (UK) Ltd, Croydon, CR0 4YY

03/10/2024

01040420-0016